Aaron Antonovsky

Health, Stress, and Coping

Jossey-Bass Publishers

San Francisco • Oxford • 1991

HEALTH, STRESS, AND COPING
New Perspectives on Mental and Physical Well-Being
by Aaron Antonovsky

Copyright © 1979 by: Jossey-Bass Inc., Publishers
350 Sansome Street
San Francisco, California 94104
&
Jossey-Bass Limited
Headington Hill Hall
London OX3 0BW

Library of Congress Catalogue Card Number LC 79-83566

International Standard Book Number ISBN 0-87589-412-7

Manufactured in the United States of America

JACKET DESIGN BY WILLI BAUM

FIRST EDITION

HB Printing   10 9 8 7 6

Code 7917

The Jossey-Bass
Social and Behavioral Science Series

For Helen
With love and gratitude

Preface

This book poses the question of *salutogenesis,* of the origins (*genesis*) of health (*saluto*). The very need for a neologism suggests that, whatever the work that has been done in this area, little of it can be called serious or systematic; the study of pathogenesis still overwhelmingly dominates medical research, whether biological or social. The book also proposes an answer to the question of salutogenesis: The origins of health are to be found in a sense of coherence. Taken together, the question and the answer are called the salutogenic model. This model, proposed by a sociologist, is, of course, only a partial conceptualization of one of the greatest mysteries in the study of people: How do we manage to stay healthy? I should like to think that the approach has sufficient cogency for it to be taken up by colleagues in other life sciences, so that some day more of the mystery is unraveled.

The book is not intended to be popular. It offers no easy solutions; as the Epilogue indicates, I tend to be a pessimist. I make no attempt to simplify a highly complex problem or to avoid technical discussion where it is necessary. The book, however, is not directed only to my major reference group, my colleagues in medical sociology. It has something to say to all those who, professionally and personally, are committed to understanding and enhancing the adaptive capacities of human beings. The professions of students in one of my seminars—sociologist, psychologist, psychiatric nurse, physician, health care organizer, epidemiologist, architect, community organizer—suggest a cross-section of my intended audience.

All advances are made by exploiting the past. I trust that those whose work has been useful to me have not been neglected in the bibliographic references. But since the book is a culmination of some fifteen years of work, as reviewed in the Introduction, I have surely borrowed from some studies without adequate acknowledgment. To their authors, my apologies. As to the works with which I should be familiar but am not, I can only plead guilty to being far from an encyclopedist.

It is appropriate to express particular indebtedness to those whose work has been of major significance for me. The responsibility is fully mine, but much of whatever merit the book has is due to what I have learned from Hans Selye, René Dubos, George Engel, and, above all, my friend and colleague Melvin Kohn.

As always, one's work is shaped and facilitated by personal contacts as well as by those whose work one has read. In this context, I must mention Abraham David Katz. Not only was David Katz a most provocative research assistant and colleague from 1968 to 1973, when many of my ideas were taking shape (Antonovsky, 1975), but more than anyone I have ever known, he embodied what I later came to call the sense of coherence. Unhappily, David Katz will never know of my gratitude; he was killed at the Suez Canal in the Yom Kippur War.

More recently, Ilana Shoham worked as my research assistant. Together with her I moved from the trees of generalized resistance resources to the forest of the sense of coherence. Ilana Shoham's brightness and critical skepticism have certainly contributed to my thinking through many problems.

The final draft of the book was written during one of the most relaxed years I have ever known, a sabbatical leave at the

School of Public Health, University of California, Berkeley. My thanks are due to Moshe Prywes, my dean at the Beersheba School of Medicine, for approving a sabbatical prior to the graduation of our first class; to Warren Winkelstein, dean of the School of Public Health, and to William Reeves, director of the Program in Epidemiology, who were my formal hosts. S. Leonard Syme, chairman of the Department of Biomedical and Environmental Health Sciences, invited me to Berkeley and, with the departmental administrative officer, Ingalill Fivian, worried about my every comfort. Because Len Syme is probably the medical sociologist whose thinking is closest to my own, I found it most useful as well as most pleasurable to have spent a year down the hall from him.

As anyone who has ever written a book knows, the cheer, intelligence, sense of humor, and efficiency of those who type and retype the manuscript are often decisive to the author's sanity. Having Constance Long and Donna Kimmel work with me was a sheer pleasure. I am truly grateful.

Among the wise decisions I have made was that to give a seminar at Berkeley devoted wholly to the manuscript of this book. These classes became a continual source of challenge for me. I did not always accept my student-colleagues' (they quickly became such) criticisms, but the need to explain why was as useful as the ideas I did take from them. My sincerest thanks, then, to Louis Allen, Margaret Boyd, Lynda Brodsky, Shoshanna Churgin, Bernard Cordes, Michael Freeman, Leslie Grant, Mario Gutierrez, Kathryn Johnson, Barbaraterry Kurtz, Eric Rosen, Barbara Sackoff, William Satariano, Sandra Stein, and Claudine Torfs.

Over the years, I have been the recipient of a number of grants, which have allowed me to pursue my work, not always as spelled out in the grant request. For these I am grateful to the United States National Institutes of Health, the Ford Foundation through the Israel Foundations Trustees, and, most recently, the Israeli Ministry of Health for its support of me as an established investigator, Chief Scientist's Bureau.

Beersheba, Israel
April 1979

AARON ANTONOVSKY

Contents

Preface   vii

The Author   xiii

Prologue: Evolution of a New Perspective   1

One   Studying Health Instead of Disease   12

Two   Measuring Health on a Continuum   38

Three Stressors, Tension, and Stress   70

Four   Tension Management and Resources for
         Resistance   98

Five   Perceiving the World as Coherent   123

Six   Relation of the Sense of Coherence to Health   160

Seven   The Salutogenic Model of Health   182

Eight   Implications for an Improved Health Care
         System   198

         Epilogue: Outlook for Human Health   220

         References   229

         Index   247

The Author

AARON ANTONOVSKY is Kunin-Lunenfeld Professor of Medical Sociology and chairman of the Department of the Sociology of Health in the Faculty of Health Services, Ben Gurion University of the Negev, Beersheba, Israel.

Antonovsky was born in Brooklyn in 1923 and attended Brooklyn College, where his undergraduate studies in history and economics were interrupted by service in the United States Army during World War II; he was awarded the B.A. degree in 1945. He did his graduate work in the Department of Sociology at Yale University, where he had his first contact with the new field of medical sociology, and was awarded the M.A. and Ph.D. degrees in sociology in 1952 and 1955, respectively. He taught evenings at Brooklyn College from 1955 to 1959, and in 1956 he became research director of the New York State Commission Against Discrimination. He was a Fulbright Professor of Sociology at the University of Teheran in 1959–1960.

With his wife Helen, a developmental psychologist, he emigrated to Israel in 1960 and accepted a post at the Israel Institute for Applied Social Research in Jerusalem, with which he is still affiliated. In the early 1960s, he began to teach in the Department of Social Medicine, and he started a research project with Judith Shuval on the latent functions of health care institutions. This project was followed by work on multiple sclerosis, coronary artery disease, menopause, preventive dental-health behavior, and early detection of cancer, as well as a series of studies on social class and various aspects of health and illness. Antonovsky spent 1965–1966 as a research fellow at the Harvard School of Public Health. In 1972, he was invited to take a central part in setting up a school of medicine at Ben Gurion University of the Negev, where he is also chairman of the Admissions Committee and where he continues his commitment to sociomedical research.

Health, Stress, and Coping

New Perspectives on Mental and Physical Well-Being

Prologue: Evolution
of a New Perspective

It is said that Oriental scholars find it appropriate to introduce their work by giving a personalized account of how they came to work on the problem and how they moved ahead, made mistakes, clarified positions, made and abandoned intellectual commitments, and finally reached the point at which they now tentatively stand. I find this approach appealing. I would like to think that, by pointing out how I came to face the issues with which I propose to deal, I can contribute clarity to the presentation. This, then, is the justification for introducing this study in somewhat autobiographical terms. Although retrospection always raises the danger of distorting the meaning experiences had when they occurred, let me nonetheless seek to retrace my steps, searching for the origins and development of my concern with what will be called salutogenesis and the sense of coherence.

1

My doctoral dissertation (Antonovsky, 1955, 1956) was not concerned explicitly with either health or psychosocial stressors. I asked how members of (what at that time was called) a minority group defined their marginal social situation. In fact, I was investigating cognitive coping responses to a socially structured psychosocial stressor. In the six years that followed, I was concerned with the same issue, though the focus shifted. Writing a history of the Jewish labor movement in the United States (Antonovsky, 1961), I dealt with the organizational response on a group level to a major nineteenth- and twentieth-century stressor, immigration. Then, as research director of the New York State Commission Against Discrimination in an era when poverty and discrimination had not quite yet been publicly discovered, I directed a number of studies on the consequences of the stressors of low income and discrimination (Antonovsky and Lorwin, 1959).

Shortly after I migrated to Israel in 1960, I became involved in a major study in the sociology of medicine, focused on the fit between "nonmedical" needs and the social structure of the health services (Shuval, Antonovsky, and Davies, 1970). At the same time, I began teaching in a school of public health. Both these projects were preliminaries to my direct entry into the field of stress research. I began collaboration with neurologists on an epidemiological study of multiple sclerosis. The literature indicated a direct correlation between distance from the equator and incidence rates. Being an anthropologically oriented sociologist, I hypothesized that societies closer to the equator differed, among other ways, from the developed societies further away in that societies closer to the equator both suffered fewer stressors and were socioculturally more competent at coping with the stressors they did face. On the basis of a relatively few items in a questionnaire, I committed myself to defining stressors objectively as those experiences that anyone anywhere would agree were stressors—for example, going hungry for extended periods. Our findings were suggestive though not definitive (Antonovsky and others, 1965; Antonovsky and Kats, 1967).

In 1965, enjoying a sabbatical at the Harvard School of Public Health, I started a series of studies that marked a continuation of my commitment to conceptualizing stressors as objective phenomena and hypothesizing a direct link between stressors and diseases. I reviewed all the empirical studies that related social class and some measure of disease. My primary concern was to bring the data together, rather than go behind the data and ask Why? (Antonovsky, 1967a, 1967b, 1968; Antonovsky and Bernstein, 1977).

During that year, however, the late John Kosa, Irving Zola, and I embarked on an editing venture that resulted in *Poverty and Health* (Kosa, Antonovsky, and Zola, 1969). In the book we asked Why? and sought to answer the question by having those writing the papers address themselves to this issue: What are the stressors in the lives of poor people that underlie the brute fact that, with regard to everything related to health, illness, and patienthood, the poor are screwed?

Ideas presented in several of the chapters, and particularly in Marc Fried's paper on mental health, marked a turning point in my thinking. Not only were the stressors important, he pointed out; but the poor also ended up badly because they had less wherewithal to battle these stressors. This marked the germination of an idea. If two people were confronted by an identical stressor, it struck me, but one had the wherewithal to successfully meet the challenge and the other did not, how could this situation best be conceptualized? Stressors by definition place a load on people. It occurred to me to call the strain incurred *tension*. The word *stress* would then be reserved for the strain that remains when the tension is not successfully overcome. The distinction compelled me to introduce a further concept, that of *tension management*, that is, the process of dealing with the tension.

I became so enthusiastic about this step forward that it came to dominate the design of my next major study. In collaboration with Ascher Segall, who had responsibility for the idea, for obtaining funding, and for doing the most complex epidemiological and medical work, I embarked on a study of the relationship between migration to Israel and coronary heart disease among North Americans (and their nonmigrant siblings). In attempting to determine whether people who migrate from a more industrialized to a less industrialized society—rare birds, indeed—have lower rates of heart disease, I included many measures of stressors in the study; but my real interest had come to be tension management and overcoming stressors (Antonovsky, 1971).

There was, however, a complication. Having abandoned stressors, so to speak, I was influenced by what has come to be known as the transactional approach. Looking back, I find confusion between saying "the impact of a given external situation upon a person is mediated by the psychological, social, and cultural resources at his disposal" (Antonovsky and Kats, 1967, p. 16) and "what is important for [the] consequences [of a life crisis] is the subjective perception of the meaning of the event rather than its objective character" (Antonovsky, 1974, p. 246). My failure to distinguish between the definition of an event as a nonstressor (suggested in the second quote) and the employment of resources to overcome an event that is defined as a stressor was not, I think, eliminated until I came to write Chapter Three in this book.

But to return to 1968. I presented a paper on the design of the coronary study at a seminar attended by the noted British epidemiologist J. N. Morris. After I had distinguished among stressor, tension, tension-management resources, and stress, Morris cogently remarked that he saw no particular reason that justified the use of the model in relation only to heart disease. It could just as reasonably (or unreasonably) be applied to any other disease. I seemed to be, he noted, interested in breakdown rather than in heart disease per se. All the way back to Jerusalem from Tel Aviv, the phrase rang in my head. It should be noted that in addition to the multiple sclerosis and coronary studies, I had also worked on a study of preventive dental-health behavior and was at the time engaged in a large-scale study of ethnic differences in adjustment to problems of climacterium. In addition, from my work on social class and health, I was familiar with a good part of the epidemiological and sociological literature on cancer, mental illness, and so on.

And then it struck me. By God, Morris is right. I am not interested in heart disease or multiple sclerosis or cancer; I am interested in breakdown. This, then, is the origin of my first major departure from the mainstream. Preparing what has come to be known as my "breakdown" paper for the Social Science and Medicine Conference in Aberdeen in 1968 (Antonovsky, 1972), I proposed a fundamental distinction between two problems: First, there is the classic problem of all of medicine: why someone gets a particular disease (or, in epidemiological terms, why a given group has a high rate of a particular disease). But, second, there is the problem of why someone gets *dis-ease* (as in John Donne's "This great hospital, this sick, this dis-easeful world"), or the problem of breakdown, whatever particular form or diagnostic category the breakdown might have.

Explicitly, I had committed myself to the idea that it was important to study breakdown as a dependent variable. I proposed an operational definition of the concept, later to be tested in the field (Antonovsky, 1973). The concept rests on the notion that there are common facets to all diseases. This definition inevitably led me to the notion of *generalized resistance resources*. Influenced by Hans Selye's concept of the general adaptation syndrome, I wrote (1972, p. 541): "Because the demands which are made on people are so variegated and in good part so unpredictable, it seems imperative to focus on developing a fuller understanding of those generalized resistance resources which can be applied to meet all demands." Further influenced by René Dubos, I began to explore the concept of adaptability in the psychological, social, and cultural spheres as one major key to successful tension management in coping with a wide variety of stressors.

At this point, then, the dependent variable that concerned me was breakdown; the independent variables were generalized resistance resources. Note that the level of stressors, objectively or subjectively defined, no longer interested me. It was quite natural for me, as a sociologist, to conceptualize breakdown, or the overall health state, as a continuum. Not being a clinician, I was not caught in the bind of categorizing people as healthy or sick. It was clear to me that all of us, as long as we are alive, are in part healthy and in part sick, that is, we are somewhere on the breakdown continuum. But "overall health state" is a misnomer. Like everyone else, I had a pathogenic orientation. (The very use of the word *breakdown* points in this direction.) My question was: What explains the fact that people move down on the breakdown continuum?

The next major step in my thinking came in the context of work on the menopause-adaptation study mentioned above. Our central interest was in the relationship between the traditionalism-modernity cultural continuum and successful adaptation to problems confronting women in the age of climacterium. Our quite large-scale study (some 1,150 women)" was based on representative samples of five ethnic groups in Israel that could reasonably be ranked on a traditionalism-modernity continuum (Datan, 1971; Datan, Antonovsky, and Maoz, forthcoming). We had good theoretical reasons for predicting a direct correlation between traditionalism and adaptation (measured in a wide variety of ways, including medical examination and location on the breakdown continuum). That is, we had reason to expect that the relatively most traditional Israeli Arab village women would be best adapted. But we had just as good reason to predict that the urban, middle-class Israeli Jewish women of Central European origin would be best adapted. I shall not reveal who on our team (a psychiatrist, a developmental psychologist, and a sociologist) took which position. But we were all right. The relation was curvilinear. The Central European women were best adapted, by and large, and close behind them came the Arab village women. The Israeli Jewish women of Turkish, North African, and Persian origin were most poorly adapted. Our post hoc analysis led to what for me was a major insight. The crucial variable in successful adaptation was not the content of culture and social structure but its relative stability. The Central European and Arab women were rooted in stable cultural contexts; the other three groups were immigrants in transition, uprooted and not yet rerooted. As will become clear, particularly in Chapter Four, this insight became a central element in my thinking about stress.

The menopause project was the stimulus for an even more fundamental turn in my thinking. For some reason that I cannot recall, we had included this question: "During World War II, were you in a concentration camp—yes or no?" Of the 287 Central European women—a representative sample of this age-sex-ethnic group taken from a middle-class Israeli community—77 said "yes." There is, in the scientific literature, almost no instance of a randomly selected sample study group compared with a control group. And we had some fourteen measures of adaptation. The results may not be surprising (Antonovsky and others, 1971): Significantly fewer of the camp survivors than of the control group were well adapted, no matter how adaptation was measured.

But then came what for me was the revolutionary question and the origin of my concern with what I only later began to call *salutogenesis*. A statistically significant difference between groups simply means that more of Group A than of Group B are high than can be accounted for by chance. It does not mean that no one in Group B is high. More than a few women among the concentration camp survivors were well adapted, no matter how adaptation was measured. Despite having lived through the most inconceivably inhuman experience, followed by Displaced Persons camps, illegal immigration to Palestine, internment in Cyprus by the British, the Israeli War of Independence, a lengthy period of economic austerity, the Sinai War of 1956, and the Six Day War of 1967 (to mention only the highlights), some women were reasonably healthy and happy, had raised families, worked, had friends, and were involved in community activities.

Other strands in my history began to be woven into the picture. Though this is meant to be an intellectual account, I cannot refrain from mentioning one personal element. My parents, now eighty-nine and eighty-three and well adapted by any standards, have not had an easy life. My father, son of a poor *shtetl* family in czarist Russia, left home at age fifteen for the city. He ran through the streets, in the midst of a raging pogrom, to call the doctor to attend my sister's birth. Illegal crossing of the border in 1921. Crossing the Atlantic in steerage three times because he and my mother did not have the right papers. Without much of a formal education, unskilled except as a Hebrew teacher, he raised a family with the "large" income, particularly during the 1930s, that came from a New York hand laundry. Mother, it is true, came from a middle-class family. But she, too, lived through all of the above and, as a woman, faced even more stressors, perhaps, than those known by a man.

Working on the second edition of *Poverty and Health,* I began groping toward the question that occurs to one when examining lives such as those of my parents: Whence the strength? Despite the fact that the poor are screwed at every step of the way, as I have put it, they are not all sick and dying. And going even further back to the 1950s, when I taught courses on "The Negroes in the United States," I recalled asking the same question about the sources of their strength. If I had previously become rather uninterested in asking people about stressors, surely doing so was superfluous for

concentration camp survivors, the poor, Afro-American slaves, or
free Negroes. (For an extremely penetrating analysis of the question
Whence the strength? see Gutman, 1976. Gutman points out that
American Negro historiography has been dominated by the question
of what slavery and subsequent conditions did to the Negro and has
seldom asked how the Negro shaped a viable culture in adapting to
the environment.) The important question, the fundamental question in scientific, humanitarian, and philosophical terms, became:
How do some of these people manage to stay reasonably healthy? I
was beginning to be freed from the pathogenic orientation. The answer, I thought, could be found by exploring generalized resistance
resources.

I am nearing the close of my story, but two major steps remain to be related. Since 1973, I have been heavily involved in the
creation of a new medical school in Israel oriented to training community primary-care physicians. I liked the idea of conceptualizing
my role in this venture, together with that of my colleagues, as
training a doctor who would be a generalized resistance resource.

While my energies were devoted largely to being a medical
school teacher, my research colleague in Jerusalem, Ilana Shoham,
was carrying out a field study that we had designed. Our dependent
variable was the breakdown continuum. Our independent variables
were an extensive series of what we thought were measures of generalized resistance resources. In the spring of 1977, shortly before I
was to leave on sabbatical, we received what is technically called a
smallest-space analysis (Guttman, 1974)—a computer printout of
the structure of relationships among a large series of variables. Lo
and behold! True, many of the resistance resources were related to
breakdown. But one resource, as we had called it, not only was more
highly correlated with our measure of overall health status, but also
seemed to be the intervening variable between the other resources
and health. For days we puzzled over the nature and meaning of
this variable, and then it clicked. This was not just another generalized resistance resource. It was a way of looking at the world. After
considering a number of alternatives, we came to call it *the sense of
coherence*.

One final step remained to be taken before I could begin
writing this book. What was to be done with stressors? As long as I

was dealing with concentration camp survivors or poor people, I could make a reasonable assumption. But what of the rest of us? Many of my colleagues in stress research are engaged in major efforts in the conceptualization and measurement of stressors. Perhaps because of my continuing interest in history since my undergraduate days or my experience as a Jew and as an Israeli or my personal peculiar combination of pessimism and optimism, it strikes me forcefully that the human condition is stressful. The question then becomes not how some concentration camp survivors or some poor people manage to stay healthy, but how *any* of us manage to stay healthy—the question of salutogenesis. I was now ready to write the book.

The central concerns of this book are, I trust, clear by now. But before we enter the detailed terrain of each chapter, in which the overall argument is inevitably obscured, let me try to provide an aerial photograph.

Chapter One spells out why salutogenesis rather than pathogenesis is the great intriguing mystery and important human concern in the field of health. The thesis is not theoretical. The hard data indicate that at any one time, at the least one third and quite possibly a majority of the population of any modern industrial society is characterized by some morbid, pathological condition, by any reasonable definition of the term. The reader who is already persuaded that illness is not at all deviant or who is willing to accept the thesis that salutogenesis is indeed at least a major issue might be content with skimming the inevitably boring statistics of the chapter.

In contrast to Chapter One, which conservatively accepts the traditional medical-model dichotomy of health and illness, Chapter Two explores the dependent variable. After reviewing the dichotomous model that is used in most health research, clinical and epidemiological, and a number of continuum models, I discuss the *health ease/dis-ease continuum,* which I see as the most appropriate tool for the study of salutogenesis.

Having set the stage, we turn to an exploration of the determinants of someone's (or some group's) location near the ease end of the continuum. Or, to put it dynamically, what explains movement toward the ease end of the continuum? Chapter Three confronts the hypothesis that the absence of, or a low level of, stressors, subjectively or objectively defined, provides the answer. This is not at all a straw man. The hypothesis lies at the basis of an entire school, in theory, in research, and in much of contemporary everyday life, of stress reduction. The evidence is overwhelming, I argue, that the hypothesis must be rejected. Stressors, I contend, are omnipresent in human existence. Further, it is important to distinguish between tension, the response of the organism to stressors, and stress, the state of the organism in response to the failure to manage tension well and to overcome stressors. Tension may even be salutary; stress is related to dis-ease.

If it is conceded that the answer to the salutogenic question lies in successful tension management, then the question becomes: What determines such success? Chapter Four suggests a tentative answer. It is based on a systematic analysis of generalized resistance resources, ranging from the physical and biochemical to the macrosociocultural. But the chapter leaves one with a nagging disquietude because of the extensive array of resources. Is there a culling rule, a theoretical basis for expecting that a given phenomenon can indeed serve as a generalized resistance resource?

Chapter Five, which answers this question, is the heart of the book. What is common to all such resources is that they facilitate making sense out of the countless stimuli with which we are constantly bombarded. Such repeated experience generates a strong sense of coherence. This central concept of the book is defined as *a global orientation that expresses the extent to which one has a pervasive, enduring though dynamic feeling of confidence that one's internal and external environments are predictable and that there is a high probability that things will work out as well as can reasonably be expected.* The bulk of the chapter is devoted to a systematic exploration of the childrearing, social-structural, and cultural sources of the generalized resistance resources that foster a strong sense of coherence. This exploration provides a link to a substantial body of work in the field that has not often been related. Finally, I review the cultural bias of locus-of-control theory, pointing up how the sense of coherence differs radically from "I am in control."

Chapter Six is devoted to a consideration of the available

evidence for the relationship between the sense of coherence and the health ease/dis-ease continuum. Since research has overwhelmingly been conducted with a pathogenic orientation and with a given disease as the dependent variable, there is a built-in limitation on the persuasibility of the argument. I hope it is sufficiently cogent to act as a stimulus for research.

The issue confronted in Chapter Seven is that of the overall structure of the salutogenic model, which is more complex than the line of argument may have suggested. Stressors are related to health, as are genetic and constitutional predispositions and weak links. Generalized resistance resources have a complex relationship to each other and to the sense of coherence. Health, in turn, is not simply a dependent variable; it is linked to well-being in other areas of life.

Chapter Eight is not necessarily an integral part of the salutogenic model. But because I am a teacher of medical students and have a deep concern for the health care of individuals and communities and because I am firmly convinced that there are implications for health care in the model, I thought it important to add this chapter. In it, I seek to spell out some of these implications, both for the relationship between the doctor (or health team) and the patient and for the organization of health care services.

Finally, in a brief Epilogue, venturing into a philosophical vein, I record the expectations that flow from the salutogenic model for the health ease of human beings in the foreseeable future. In doing so, I compare and contrast my views with the optimistic ones of Lewis Thomas, the on-balance optimistic views of Thomas McKeown, the on-balance pessimistic views of René Dubos, and the pessimism of Ivan Illich.

Chapter One

Studying Health Instead of Disease

The problem of salutogenesis is one of the most mysterious, intriguing, and meaningful challenges for philosophy and the biological and the social sciences. Pathogenesis—the origins of disease X, disease Y, disease Z—has preoccupied us (to the extent that we have focused on origins and not only on diagnosis and therapy). Even immunology, the science perhaps most closely linked to salutary, homeostasis-maintaining and homeostasis-restoring processes, has posed its questions largely in terms palatable to pathogenesis: What will prevent this or that disease? I hope it will become clear in due course that my concern is no mere semantic quibble and that here, as in all of science, how one poses the question is crucial to the direction one takes in looking for the answers.

I had considered using the term *orthogenesis,* the origins of being straight or upright. The term, however, has been preempted by others and generally refers to treatment aimed at correcting mental and nervous defects in children. *Eugenics,* too, which concerns improvement of the human race by mating, is not an apt term for the concept I propose to develop. Since my concern is not primarily with issues of repairing or straightening out (though a theory of salutogenesis certainly bears important implications for orthogenics) nor with improvement through mating, I have opted for a neologism—*salutogenesis.*

To ask why someone gets viral pneumonia or hypertensive heart disease or a fractured rib or schizophrenia or any one of the 1,040 major morbid conditions listed in the International Statistical Classification of Diseases, Injuries, and Causes of Death is to ask a difficult scientific and clinically important question. There is no end to the basic and subsequently applied research needed to elucidate the complex hundreds of answers. Commitment to such activity, however, tends to lead to what Dubos (1960)' has argued is a commitment to an illusion. To think that conquering one disease after another brings us that much closer to conquering disease in general has double-edged consequences. On the one hand, it provides the motivation, courage, and resources for societies and people to devote themselves to the struggle of understanding and coping with real problems and real human suffering. On the other hand, it dulls our sensitivity to and concern with some painfully hard morbidity data in the second half of the twentieth century. Moreover, it inevitably diverts attention and resources from the real mystery and from what I shall contend is the most promising direction to take in attempting to make our life better.

Let me put it bluntly. Given the ubiquity of pathogens—microbiological, chemical, physical, psychological, social, and cultural—it seems to me self-evident that everyone should succumb to this bombardment and constantly be dying. Dubos (1965, p. 35) has highlighted the solution to part of the problem as "the control of the disease states caused by microbial agents which are ubiquitous in our communities in the form of dormant infections." Before the public health triumphs in controlling sanitation, food, and water; before the generally improved standards of living, particularly of nutrition; before the discoveries of medical microbiology and pharmacology, acute and semiacute infectious processes were caused largely by microorganisms acquired through exposure to an exogenous source of infection. These pathogens have hardly disappeared, even from the Western world, but they can largely be controlled or, at least, their consequences can be contained. There are problems of drug-resistant strains of pathogenic agents and social problems of application of existing knowledge and techniques. But the major infectious diseases in the Western world are now related to the omnipresent, endogenous microorganisms that make the event of infection much less important than the smoldering infectious process.

There are, then, the descendants of the exogenous "bugs" that have been of such great significance in human history (Burnet, 1953). There are the endogenous bugs, whose virulence may be held in abeyance but whose threat is constant. There are, third, those agents, be they viruses, mutant cells, pollutants, or agents of physical trauma such as guns, knives, and motor vehicles, that pose a constant threat of damage, reparable or irreparable, immediately evident or slowly unfolding, to the human organism. And, finally, there are those bugs variously called psychosocial stressors, presses, strains: alienation, rapid social change, identity crises, ends-means gaps, discrimination, anxiety, frustration. I shall, in Chapter Three, discuss the issue of psychosocial stressors in some detail. But for the time being, and in full awareness of the complexity, softness, speculativeness, and even problems of elementary definition in viewing psychosocial stressors as pathogens, I would maintain that there is sufficient ground for including them in this litany of bugs.

In sum, it seems to me that elementary knowledge and observation of the world around us must inevitably raise the question of how anyone ever stays alive. The human capacity for consciousness, for taking in this miserably hostile world—its glories and wonders notwithstanding—must certainly lead us to ponder the ultimate mystery of salutogenesis. Surely, the reader must respond, I have exaggerated. Even casual observation suggests that most of us, most of the time, are not on our deathbeds, are not in the hospital, and are more or less healthy. The world around us cannot be as virulent as I have suggested; or at least we have learned to live in some balance with the world so that we do not succumb that often to the bugs. What are the facts?

I shall, in Chapter Two, deal in some detail with the question of what sickness, disease, ill health, or health is. I shall there argue that it makes the most sense to picture the answers on a complex, multidimensional continuum. I see little utility in a dichotomous classification of sick-well, pathological-salutological. But for the present, I shall consider data that deal with conditions that would be considered pathological or morbid in the orthodox medical model.

Morbidity Hypothesis

My contention can be put in a straightforward manner. At any one time, at least one third and quite possibly a majority of the population of any modern industrial society is characterized by some morbid condition, by any reasonable definition of the term. Or, to put it another way, deviance, clinically or epidemiologically defined, is "normal." That is, significant departures from the clinical picture of health are, statistically, far from unusual.

One would think that, having formulated this hypothesis on the basis of the theoretical consideration that bugs are ubiquitous, one could easily test it. All one need do is turn to any textbook of epidemiology and find a distribution of the population as having no morbid condition; one morbid condition, with subclassification; two or more morbid conditions, with subclassification. A search of six standard texts revealed no such table or reference to the issue. I then examined the vast repository of data put out by the U.S. National Center for Health Statistics on the basis of the National Health Survey. Again, my efforts were largely in vain. In sum, I found no single source that could provide sufficiently detailed evidence to test the hypothesis. Oral inquiries to epidemiologists confirmed this lack of data; moreover, they not only noted the methodological difficulties in obtaining such a set of data but were usually surprised that the question was raised (see Morris, 1957, p. 11).

That this is the case should not have surprised me, for it bears out the point I wish to make. Our dominant ideological paradigm, which shapes our society's clinical practice and scientific research, focuses on and responds to a particular disease or clinical entity. Our health care system, or, as Winkelstein (1972) has cogently suggested, our disease care system, focuses on individual diseases. But even those such as Winkelstein who urge more attention to health care still set problems in terms of pathogenesis: how to prevent lung cancer, motor vehicle accidents, or poliomyelitis. Hence data are most often collected on cases of specific disease rather than on the location of people on a health-disease continuum or even in an overall category of morbidity. We somehow assume that most people are healthy because we focus on individual diseases. Even so revolutionary a thinker as Dubos, who perhaps more than anyone else first set me on the path I now tread in teaching us of the mirage of health, thinks largely of specific diseases. Only when we begin to pose the problem of salutogenesis will we begin to fully implement a full-scale search for those factors that promote health rather than cause specific diseases.

Morbidity Data

The problem of salutogenesis, however, emerges in its full significance only when we look at the data. It is to these that I now turn. It is not my purpose, nor would it have been possible, to arrive at a definitive set of data that would adequately answer the question: At any one time, how many people are (or what part of the population is) characterized by explicit, significant morbid conditions? I have set as my limited goal to submit the contention presented above to a rough but fair test of empirical data. I have tried to err on the conservative side. I leave it to the reader, given the data and their sources, to judge the extent to which the contention is supported.

Since this book was written in the United States, the data most easily available to me were those that refer to that country. My purpose not being epidemiological, I have not considered it important to present relevant data from other Western countries. They have been reviewed and unhappily show a similar picture. For the most recent published survey available to me, see the work of Bridges-Webb (1973, 1974) on a small Australian community. It seems quite safe to say that data on nonindustrialized societies would show a far bleaker picture.

Let us start from a 1961 statement by White, Williams, and

Greenberg: "Data from medical care studies in the United States and Great Britain suggest that in a population of 1,000 adults (sixteen years of age and over) in an average month 750 will experience an episode of illness and 250 of these will consult a physician." No doubt many of the 250 who do come to the doctor are not what, by medical consensus at least, would be called ill; there is equally no doubt that many among the 500 who experience an illness episode but do not go to the doctor are not what, again by medical consensus, we would call ill. But we must add that there may well be some among the 250 without an episode of illness who can conservatively be called ill. (We are not here concerned with the extremely important issue of going to the doctor—an issue that these data raise.) These data led Zola (1966, p. 616) to conclude that "the empirical reality may be that illness, defined as the presence of clinically serious symptoms, is the statistical norm."

Chronic Illness. To the best of my knowledge, only one published study comes close to adequately documenting the requisite data, and we would do best to start from it, even though it is limited to one urban community. Moreover, the Baltimore study of the Commission on Chronic Illness (1957) focuses, as the name indicates, on one element (chronic illness) of the picture, albeit the most important one. But before considering the Baltimore study, we should keep in mind one fact noted by the authors of that study. Neither it nor other studies based on fieldwork include institutionalized persons. In 1970, some 1,670,100 persons were in long-term-care institutions for clearly nonhealthy people, a prevalence rate of 828/100,000. This figure includes those in mental and tuberculosis hospitals, nursing homes, and homes and schools for the mentally and physically handicapped (National Center for Health Statistics, 1976). (For data on the health status of nursing home residents, see National Center for Health Statistics, 1977b.) This figure excludes all persons in correctional institutions, detention homes, homes for neglected children and unwed mothers—settings that are likely to contain a higher proportion of sick people (by age group) than do noninstitutional settings. Moreover, the data show a marked decline in numbers compared with the data for the previous decade, largely because of the substantial decline of people in mental institutions.

It is not my purpose here to go into details in a critical review of the Baltimore study or any of the other data presented since it is totally out of the question to do anything more than obtain rough approximations of the proportions of the population who are ill. Suffice it to say that the Baltimore data are based on a representative citywide sample of 11,574 persons. The Baltimore of the mid 1950s differed in one major respect from some other large cities in its large (27 percent) nonwhite population, a fact that would tend to be reflected in somewhat more chronic illness than might be found in other cities. Keeping this in mind, we turn to the data.

The prevalence rate of chronic diseases in the city of Baltimore in 1954 was 156,650/100,000 persons, or almost 1.6 diseases per person (p. 50). Almost two thirds (64.9 percent) of the population had a chronic condition, a proportion that varied from almost 30 percent of those under fifteen to 95 percent of those over sixty-five. (See pp. 393–399 of the study for a definition of chronic condition.) When reference is made to substantial chronic conditions—"those which interfered with or limited the patient's activities or were likely to do so in the future, or which required or were likely to require care"—the proportion of the population so characterized fell to 44.4 percent: 19 percent with one substantial condition, 13 percent with two, and 12 percent with three or more (pp. 55–56). A classification of the conditions as mild, moderate, or severe in the present stage showed that only one eighth of the conditions were severe (as indicated by an increasing degree of disabling effects, a more advanced state of the disease, a greater likelihood of fatality, a need for more care, complications, or increasing pain). But this qualification would seem to be unduly sanguine in light of the detailed classification found in Table 1.

A second (albeit secondary and not recent) source of data on chronic diseases in the United States is Blum and Keranen's authoritative review (1966). Following the definition of chronic disease formulated by the authors of the Baltimore study, they estimate that 42 percent of the population suffers from one or more chronic conditions. Blum and Keranen most often do not give rates. Where they do, they are by and large comparable to the Baltimore findings. Thus, for example, they estimate that about 2 percent of the population has diabetes (p. 145) compared with Baltimore's 2.67. Similarly, 2 percent are estimated to have no functional hearing (p. 30), the same proportion found for deafness and impaired hearing in the Baltimore study. Where Blum and Keranen differ, they tend to have somewhat higher estimates than the rates found in Baltimore. Thus "asthma affects about 2½ percent of the U.S. population" (p. 35) compared with Baltimore's 1.24 percent.

Blum and Keranen also speak of "an estimated two million survivors of stroke" (p. 265); anemia in "4 to 15 percent of the adult population, depending upon the hemoglobin level defined as abnormal" (p. 71); and "hyperuricemia is estimated to affect approximately 3 percent of the U.S. population" (p. 108).

Finally, Blum and Keranen classify as chronic a number of conditions that are not covered in the Baltimore study and that are of widespread significance. Among these are diseases of the bronchopulmonary system, such as chronic bronchitis, "estimated to affect between 15 and 20 percent of persons over forty in both the United States and England" (p. 37), and pulmonary emphysema, which affects "about 12 percent of adult males" (p. 40); and alcoholism, found among "nearly 5 percent of adults" (p. 153).

A more recent and comprehensive review of the data is found in a publication of an authoritative, respectable body (National Health Education Committee, 1976). The data must, however, be taken with some caution since they are assembled mainly from organizations in the medical-research and medical-service establishment, whose vested interest is reflected in a possible overestimate of prevalence rates. This issue is dealt with later in this chapter, but it is of sufficient import to be noted at this point. I should add that the estimates presented do not differ greatly from those from other sources.

As seen in Table 2, in which the data on the main causes of disability in the United States are presented, there is a total of about 108 million cases of these morbid conditions. This is about 52 percent of the total population. There is of course overlap. Individuals who have multiple conditions are counted as two or possibly more cases. Thus, the estimated 30.33 million cases of the four major circulatory diseases included in the table (high blood pressure, coronary heart disease, rheumatic heart disease, and strokes) are found among 27.13 million persons, an overlap that is perhaps surprisingly low. There is no way of estimating how many individuals, in all, are afflicted by these 108 million conditions.

Included in this list are 6 million mentally retarded, 11.5

Table 1. Prevalence of Chronic Diseases, Baltimore, 1954

Diagnosis	Rate per 100,000 Persons
ALL DIAGNOSES	156,650
Other diseases of female genital organs	13,360[a]
Obesity	12,890
Heart disease	9,640
Arthritis	7,520
Hypertension without heart involvement	6,640
Neoplasms (of which malignant or unspecified—300)	5,490
Hemorrhoids	5,370
Psychoneuroses	5,260
Diseases of prostate	4,440[a]
Varicose veins of lower extremities	4,370
Cervicitis	4,350[a]
Hernia of abdominal cavity	3,660
Psychophysiological autonomic and visceral disorders	3,650
Syphilis	3,650
Orthopedic impairments not elsewhere classified (except cerebral paralysis)	3,380
Low back strain	3,010
Diabetes mellitus	2,670
Anemia	2,600
Diseases of thyroid	2,460
Deafness and impaired hearing	2,000
Hay fever	1,750
Cataract (not causing blindness)	1,720

million people with hearing impairments, and 9.6 million people with visual impairments. A conservative approach would exclude most, though by no means all, of these persons from a count of the type we are attempting here. However, Table 2 does not include data on diseases that are covered in the text of the source. Thus, for example, "about 17 percent of the total population are estimated to suffer from an allergy at any given time" (p. 6); of this total, about 11 percent have asthma or hay fever or both. "Approximately 1,306,000 have such severe visual impairment that they are unable to read ordinary newsprint with either eye, even with glasses" (p. 34)—a rate of about 625/100,000; the condition is caused mainly by retinal diseases, glaucoma, or cataract. About 475,000

Table 1. Prevalence of Chronic Diseases, Baltimore, 1954 (cont'd)

Diagnosis	Rate per 100,000 Persons
Other mental, psychoneurotic, and personality disorders	1,520
Diseases of gall bladder	1,370
Arteriosclerosis	1,290
Other diseases of circulatory system	1,290
Asthma	1,240
Other allergies	1,160
Symptoms referable to limbs and back	1,110
Chronic sinusitis	880
Migraine	750
Tuberculosis	630
Blindness and impaired vision	610
Cerebral paralysis not elsewhere classified	610
Other diseases of central nervous system	580
Psychoses	430
Diseases of kidney	360
Vascular lesions of central nervous system	260
Rheumatic fever without heart involvement	40
Other symptoms, senility, and ill-defined causes	5,080
All other diagnoses	38,280

Note: Since some rates are sex-specific, the overall rate for all diagnoses is less than the sum of all the detailed rates.

a Sex-specific disease.

Source: Commission on Chronic Illness (1957, pp. 527–529).

persons are blind by legal criteria (228/100,000). "Approximately two million Americans lack sufficient hearing to understand speech" (p. 93). Acute and chronic digestive diseases (disorders of the stomach, intestines, biliary passages, liver, and pancreas) "affect about thirteen million Americans" (p. 105). "An estimated fifteen million Americans today suffer the consequences of birth defects of varying severity," of which about 20 percent are the effects of damage to the fetus and 80 percent are true genetic diseases; this estimate does not include conditions suspected of having a genetic component— for example, schizophrenia—or the 10 to 12 percent of the population with enzyme or other deficiencies often involved in adverse

Table 2. Main Causes of Disability, United States, Early 1970s

Condition	Prevalence Rate per 100,000[a]	Number of People Afflicted to Some Degree (in Millions)
High blood pressure	11,053	23.0
Arthritis and rheumatic diseases	9,707	20.2
Mental and emotional disorders (in some degree)	9,611	20.0
Hearing impairments	5,527	11.5
Visual impairments	4,612	9.596
Mental retardation	2,883	6.0
Coronary heart disease	1,941	4.04
Diabetes mellitus	1,922	4.0
Epilepsy	1,442	2–4.0
Rheumatic heart disease	803	1.67
Cerebrovascular disease (strokes)	779	1.62
Cancer (under medical care now)	493	1.025
Parkinsonism	481	1.0
Cerebral palsy	360	0.75
Multiple sclerosis and related diseases	240	0.5
Muscular dystrophy	96	0.2

[a] The prevalence estimates in the source are given in absolute numbers and refer to somewhat different years. I have calculated the rates on the basis of the 1973 population (208,087,000), which gives a somewhat larger denominator and hence a lower rate for most conditions.

Source: National Health Education Committee (1976, p. 291).

drug reactions, nor does it reflect the data on spontaneous abortions (pp. 121–123). "About nine million people in the United States today are alcoholics and alcohol abusers" (p. 153). "There were in the United States, in 1970, 294,000 active and arrested cases of tuberculosis," of which 157,000 were active cases (p. 250).

Specific Chronic Diseases and Impairments. Data for a few selected chronic diseases are found in *Health: United States, 1975* (National Center for Health Statistics, 1976). These rates (per 100,000), too, are generally consistent with those above: arthritis— 9,290; asthma—3,020; chronic bronchitis—3,270; and diabetes— 2,040 (p. 247).

The Baltimore study found a prevalence rate of 270 for *malignant neoplasms* and 30 for neoplasms of unspecified nature.

This is, however, surely an underestimation. According to the estimate of the American Cancer Society (see Table 2), "more than one million people were under medical care for cancer in 1975." In 1974, a total of 655,000 new cases were reported, excluding carcinoma in situ of the uterine cervix and superficial skin cancers, which are unlikely to be reported. Given the fact that malignant neoplasms are the primary cause of about 18 percent of all deaths and that, roughly, the overall five-year cancer survival rate is about 40 percent today, I have calculated that the prevalence rate of cancer is likely to be in the neighborhood of 800/100,000. This estimate is consistent with the incidence data given in the second and third National Cancer Study reports (Dorn and Cutler, 1959, p. 13; Cutler and Young, 1975, pp. 307–342) and is lower than the rate given in Levin and others (1974, p. 4).

Estimates of the prevalence of selected *chronic circulatory conditions* in the United States in 1972 were arrived at on the basis of a national sample of 44,000 households in the Health Interview Survey (National Center for Health Statistics, 1974). Rates per 100,000 persons range from 6,010 for hypertensive disease, 5,040 for heart conditions, 4,770 for hemorrhoids, and 3,680 for varicose veins to 750 for cerebrovascular disease, 440 for congenital anomalies of the circulatory system, and 160 for phlebitis and thrombophlebitis. On the basis of a number of methodological studies comparing interview reports with examination results, the report concludes—in accord with all studies on the subject—that interview data provide considerable underestimation of the prevalence of chronic conditions (see Feldman, 1960). The extent, of course, varies considerably from condition to condition. Bearing in mind this underestimation in interview data, we still find over forty-four million chronic circulatory conditions estimated. Again, one must take note of duplication. The report estimates that these conditions were found among 36,492,000 persons, or 17.7 percent of the U.S. population. Of these, over 26,000,000 were under age sixty-five. Obviously, conditions with a wide range of severity and impact are included here. But even a conservative approach cannot dismiss the existence of varicose veins as a morbid condition even though in only 3.9 percent of the cases were varicose veins reported as having caused some limitation of activity during the year.

A somewhat earlier report in the Health Interview Survey

indicates the prevalence of fifteen selected *chronic respiratory conditions* in 1970 (National Center for Health Statistics, 1973b). Again, the prevalence rates vary greatly: from 10,300/100,000 for chronic sinusitis and 5,420 for hay fever to only 60 for pneumoconiosis. Also, chronic bronchitis (3,270) and emphysema (660)' suggest far different prognoses than does a deflected nasal septum (400). Nonetheless, if we project these figures to the total U.S. civilian, noninstitutionalized population, we can estimate a total of 53,754,000 conditions distributed among 46,884,000 people, of whom almost 42,000,000 are under sixty-five.

The third in the series of National Center for Health Statistics (1973a) studies of chronic morbidity that merits reference here reports on *chronic digestive conditions*. The ten condition groups reviewed in this 1968 survey (for example, ulcer of the stomach and duodenum, a rate of 1,720; gall bladder condition, 1,030; chronic enteritis and ulcerative colitis, 930) are projected to almost twenty-one million conditions in the country, affecting a total of seventeen million people, of whom 4,610,000 are sixty-five and over.

Finally, we may take note of a 1971 survey of the prevalence of *impairments* that have merited listing in the International Classification of Diseases. The impairments reviewed range from hearing impairments, which have a rate of 7,160 (of which only 4 percent cause limitation of activity), to complete or partial paralysis, with a rate of 690 (with 62 percent of the conditions causing limitation of activity). In all, some 47.4 million conditions included here are found in the United States, affecting 37.3 million persons, of whom 9.8 percent are sixty-five and over (National Center for Health Statistics, 1975).

Two major chronic conditions have largely been ignored. The disease known as *dental caries* is, as Blum and Keranen put it (1966, p. 76), universal. "Very few people," they add, "escape some degree of gingivitis or periodontal disease." Whether it is because historically medicine and dentistry have gone their separate ways or because dental disease is not a cause of mortality among humans (in contrast to animals) or perhaps because of their near universality, such problems are not often referred to in discussions of chronic diseases. Yet if one's criterion is suffering, then surely this must be one of the major areas demanding attention, and it certainly cannot be neglected in this review of the data.

The second area, that of *mental retardation* and *mental illness,* has been mentioned. My own preference is to exclude mental retardation from a discussion of chronic disease. Although 3 percent of the population scores below 70 on nationally standardized intelligence tests, the overwhelming majority of such persons are, I am persuaded, not to be included within the scope of a conservatively oriented discussion of disease problems. No more than 100 per 100,000 persons—a far cry from the 2,883 rate cited in Table 2— are the legitimate concern of the disease care institution. I do not, of course, in any way mean that mental retardation is not a major problem of social concern. I am saying that it is not, in the main, a medical problem. Many persons classified as mentally retarded, appropriately or not, indeed come to the attention of the disease care institution, but this is a totally different issue from the one that concerns us at present.

Mental illness, however, cannot be excluded from this discussion. I am persuaded that Szasz and his colleagues and the labeling theorists in medical sociology have made a major contribution in compelling us to confront the meaning of mental illness (Szasz, 1963; Becker, 1963; Goffman, 1961; Scheff, 1966; see Gove, 1970, for a critique). But I cannot accept their position that mental illness is not a legitimate concern of the health care or disease care institution. It would take us too far afield to consider the various arguments and to support my position here. Suffice it to say that I am fully aware of and indebted to Szasz and the others and seek to err on the side of caution in considering the data.

The data suggest that few indeed are the adults who have always been free of significant emotional symptoms. But Susser notes, "The fact that the presence of symptoms is the norm in a population does not necessarily rule out their pathological significance" (1968, pp. 208–214). Being somewhat less inclusive, we take note of the Midtown Manhattan study, which found that 23 percent of the community sample suffered mental impairment from symptoms classified as marked, severe, or incapacitating (Srole and others, 1962). Susser, judiciously reviewing the evidence available, suggests—as I read him—a true prevalence rate of severe psychiatric illness ranging from 1,000 to 3,000 per 100,000 adults below age sixty, the rate being somewhat higher among older persons.

Finally, in this review of chronic-disease data, we turn to the category of *allergy*. We do best by quoting from a popular but highly reliable source (Roueche, 1978, p. 63) : "Allergy differs from most other diseases in that its victims (including even most asthmatics) seldom die and almost as seldom recover. . . . Allergy is, . . . in fact, the most common of all chronic complaints throughout the industrially developed world. . . . The allergic population of the United States is on the way to forty million. Almost fifteen million of these are hay fever sufferers. Nine million are asthmatic, and another several million are allergic to some food or drug or drink. The rest . . . are victims of allergic eczematous contact dermatitis."

Notifiable Diseases. We now turn to a different categorization of diseases, which cuts across the above-considered chronic diseases and the soon-to-be-considered acute conditions—that is, specified notifiable diseases that are under the egis of the Center for Disease Control. In 1977, a total of eighteen cases of plague were reported in the United States, four of cholera, and none of smallpox or yellow fever. But unlike these diseases, which are covered by international quarantine agreement and which seem, for the time being, to have come close to having been eradicated in the United States, there are other communicable diseases whose incidence is not negligible. For the present purposes, these would not include such diseases as anthrax, botulism, brucellosis, diphtheria, leprosy, leptospirosis, malaria, meningococcal infections, poliomyelitis, psittacosis, rabies in man, congenital rubella syndrome, tetanus, trichinosis, tularemia, typhoid fever, typhus fever, and venereal diseases other than syphilis and gonorrhea. (I have quite intentionally included this long list of diseases, none of which has yet been removed from the list of notifiable diseases, as a reminder that secular trends in disease prevalence are not necessarily, as liberal ideology would have it, unidirectional.)

Those notifiable diseases that have annual incidence rates of 10 or higher per 100,000 are contained in Table 3. The rates for all but gonorrhea seem to be quite modest. Clearly, compared with the chronic diseases, these morbid conditions are of relatively minor

Table 3. Reported Cases of Specified Notifiable Diseases,
United States, 1977

Disease	Annual Incidence Rate per 100,000	Number of Cases
Gonorrhea[a]	465.9	1,000,177
Chickenpox	97.6	188,396
Syphilis[a]	30.0	64,473
Measles (rubeola)	26.5	57,345
Hepatitis	26.2	56,623
Tuberculosis	13.9	30,145
Salmonellosis, excluding typhoid fever	12.9	27,850
Mumps	10.0	21,436

[a] Newly reported civilian cases.

Source: Center for Disease Control (September 1978, pp. 2, 3).

significance in scope. Tuberculosis and diphtheria are no longer among the ten leading causes of death. Thus, for present purposes, and for the population as a whole, relatively little contribution is made by these communicable diseases to overall morbidity; the number of reported cases of somewhat under 1.5 million, even assuming no overlap at all, is small compared with the number of cases of other morbid conditions. Yet note must be taken of the not thoroughly investigated problem of stigma in reporting. "When underreporting and undetected cases are considered, it is estimated that about two million cases of gonorrhea occur each year . . . and that about 450,000 persons are in need of treatment for syphilis (includes all stages) at the present time" (National Center for Health Statistics, 1976, p. 258). This, in contrast with the one million new cases of gonorrhea and 64,000 new cases of syphilis that were reported in 1977.

Acute Conditions. We now turn to acute conditions, for which, by their very nature, it is next to impossible to establish prevalence rates. Further, reporting or not reporting acute conditions in a survey is strongly influenced by cultural and social-structural as well as by psychological factors. These caveats notwithstanding, I believe some approximations are possible. The National

Health Survey, our major source of data, defines an acute morbidity condition as a reported "departure from a state of physical or mental well-being . . . which has lasted less than three months and which has involved either medical attention or restricted activity" (National Center for Health Statistics, 1978, p. 57); chronic conditions are thus excluded. The data are classified in five condition groups, following the International Classification of Diseases: infective and parasitic diseases, respiratory conditions, digestive-system conditions, injuries, and all other acute conditions (ear disorders, headaches, genitourinary disorders, skin disorders, and so forth).

In the year July 1975–June 1976, every man, woman, and child in the United States had more than two episodes, on the average, of an acute illness or injury requiring medical attention or restriction of usual daily activity (an annual incidence of 214,300/100,000). The detailed data on the incidence and duration of these acute conditions are contained in Table 4.

Clearly, acute conditions vary greatly in seriousness and personal or social implications. On the one hand, the list includes the common cold (accounting for 20.7 percent of all acute conditions) and sprains and strains (3.4 percent); on the other hand, it includes pneumonia (0.8 percent) and genitourinary disorders (2.6 percent). Bearing in mind that the evidence points to substantial underreporting of acute conditions as well, even in a two-week recall period as is the case here, we can clearly see that the 450 million estimated episodes of acute conditions in one year form part of the record. Using the data contained in Table 4, I have calculated that on any given day, almost 2.6 percent of the population had an acute illness or injury (average number of restricted-activity days multiplied by 365).

Disability and Limitation. Having raised the issue of the impact of illness or injury on disability or activity limitation, I will pursue the issue further in order to look at our basic question— How many people are ill at any given time? —from another point of view. Again using the data of the National Health Survey (National Center for Health Statistics, 1977a), we find that in 1976 the average American had 18.2 restricted-activity days—days on which he or she substantially reduced normal activity for the whole day because of an illness, either chronic or acute, or an injury. This fig-

Table 4. Annual Incidence Rates and Impact of Acute Conditions, United States, July 1975–June 1976

Condition Group	Annual Incidence per 100,000	Average Duration of Disability (Days)		Days per 100 Persons per Year	
		Restricted Activity	Bed Disability	Restricted Activity	Bed Disability
ALL ACUTE CONDITIONS	214,300	4.4	2.0	939.2	422.4
Infective and parasitic diseases	23,800	4.0	2.2	94.4	51.5
Respiratory conditions	115,100	3.6	1.9	418.8	218.6
Digestive-system conditions	9,900	4.4	2.2	43.1	21.9
Injuries	33,600	6.3	1.8	213.3	59.3
All other	31,800	5.3	2.2	169.6	71.1

Source: National Center for Health Statistics (1978, pp. 5, 11, 12).

ure does not include persons who have permanently reduced their usual activities because of a chronic condition; the data refer only to those who had a reduced level of activity within the two-week period prior to the interview compared with the level of activity before that period. The number of restricted-activity days averages around 11 per year per person under age twenty-five, 15.5 for persons twenty-five to forty-four, 25.4 for persons forty-five to sixty-four, and 40 for persons sixty-five years and over.

The same source provides another way of looking at the direct, reported consequences of chronic conditions in the data on limitation of activity. Setting up criteria appropriate to children, housekeepers, workers, and others, the Health Interview Survey found that on the day of the interview, in 1976, 14.3 percent of the population had some limitation of usual activity due to a chronic condition. It is true that this situation is particularly characteristic of elderly persons (45.4 percent of those sixty-five and over), but it is also true of 24.3 percent of those forty-five to sixty-four years old. Moreover, if only one's major activity is considered, 10.8 percent of the total population reported a limitation. This proportion rises to 19.1 percent of those aged forty-five to sixty-four.

In considering these figures, one should keep in mind that all these data refer to the civilian, noninstitutionalized population. Earlier, we referred to the likelihood that some 0.8 percent of the population are, at one time, in long-term institutions for sick people. At this point it is appropriate to add that the surveys also do not include people who, at the time of the survey, were in short-stay hospitals. During 1976 there were an estimated 14,100 hospital discharges per 100,000 persons. The average length of stay was 7.9 days. Or, to put it another way, about 10.6 percent of the population was hospitalized at least once during the year preceding the interview in the Health Interview Survey. This figure does not include persons who died in the hospital, but it does include hospital deliveries (National Center for Health Statistics, 1977a).

Overall Morbidity. In closing my review of the data, I refer to two studies of morbidity without detailed consideration of specific pathologies. Chapter Two deals with this problem conceptually; for the time being, I refer to the issue only to test the hypothesis posed initially in this chapter. In 1965 a probability sample of 6,928 adult residents of Alameda County, California, completed questionnaires that used four central measures: ability to perform certain basic daily activities; presence during the previous year of one or more chronic conditions or impairments; presence during the previous year of one or more symptoms; and subjective rating of general energy level. On the basis of the detailed responses to this set of questions, respondents were placed on a seven-category ordinal scale, ranging from severe disability to high energy level (Belloc, Breslow, and Hochstim, 1971).

Of the total sample, representing a community of some one million adults, 29 percent were classified in the no-complaint categories (23 percent low to medium energy, 6 percent high energy). At the other extreme, 7 percent reported a severe disability, an additional 8 percent a lesser disability, 9 percent two or more chronic conditions, 19 percent one chronic condition, and 28 percent at least one symptom. There were, of course, sharp differences by age. If a cutting point of at least one chronic condition is used (that is, including the four poorer categories and excluding symptoms), we find 43 percent of the population included, ranging from about one fifth of the youngest age group, through close to half of those aged forty-five to fifty-four, to over three fourths of those sixty-five and over. What should be stressed is that the no-complaint–high-energy group remained almost constant at 6 or 7 percent in all age groups through ages sixty-five to seventy-four and then dropped to 4 percent.

In contrast to the first study, whose major goal was to obtain an epidemiological picture of the health status of a community, the study reported by Collen (1977) presents data assembled in the context of multiphasic screening in a prepaid health care plan organization. Data are given on 6,285 adults who had not seen a physician within one year and who asked for a multiphasic checkup. Thus, on the one hand, these persons evidently felt well enough to go without seeing a doctor for a year; on the other hand, they had some motivation for having the checkup. We have no way of knowing how representative the group was of a total community population; certainly there is no reason to think that the error was on the side of being unduly ill. (In a personal communication, Collen informed me that Kaiser data show that persons who come for multiphasics have been found to be healthier than a control group of members who do not come.) Recall, too, that they were members of a prepaid health care plan. Those classified as well (no significant medical complaint or problem and no clinically significant finding or abnormality) constituted 56.8 percent; worried-well (complaint but no finding), 11.6 percent; asymptomatic-sick (no complaint but clinically significant finding), 3.9 percent; and sick (both complaint and finding), 27.7 percent. Thus sick care, within this organization, was needed for 32 percent.

Methodological Considerations. Before we consider the significance of the data for the central concern of this book, it is appropriate to make a number of methodological comments. First, I would reiterate the issue of overlap, which has been mentioned in passing a number of times. Individuals who contribute to the numerator in one rate may also contribute to the numerator in another rate. For example, our point of departure, the Baltimore study, reported an average of 1.6 chronic conditions per person. Yet, as noted with regard to the discussion of cardiovascular diseases, this overlap is not always as great as one might think. Unfortunately, the pathogenic orientation, which focuses on specific diseases, has prevented any possibility of a firm conclusion on the question of overlap. It may well be that many older people have multiple conditions. But, as the data on disability and activity limitation as well as the Health Interview Survey reports indicate, those under sixty-five do not present a picture of blooming health.

A second issue to be noted is conceptual confusion—in part inevitable—of risk factors, pathology, and consequences. I have tried to limit this confusion without forfeiting data. Thus, I mentioned alcoholism and obesity but not smoking. Only cultural definitions legitimate referring to alcoholism and obesity as morbid or pathological. In all likelihood, smoking is more implicated in mortality than is either alcoholism or obesity, yet somehow our medical culture regards alcoholism and obesity as pathological but sees smoking only as a risk factor. In the same vein, note should be taken that I make no mention of accidents, suicide, or homicide (respectively, the third, ninth, and tenth causes of death in the United States in 1973, considering all cardiovascular diseases jointly; see National Health Education Committee, 1976, p. 289). Accidents and violence are causes of morbid conditions, however, and hence presumably are reflected in the data on pathology.

The third issue that affects the reliability of the rates of morbidity reported here is that of the "iceberg" phenomenon so well known to epidemiologists—that is, the gap between the "true" prevalence—if only we were able to count every truly existent case, whatever that may mean with regard to a given morbid condition—and the reported or counted prevalence. To what extent this factor has led to the data presented being underestimates cannot be known. It is appropriate that the issue be mentioned; but there is, I believe, no need to consider it in evaluating the extent to which the hypothesis of the chapter is supported by the data.

No doubt, however, vested interests have, to some extent, overestimated the prevalence of pathology, a fourth consideration. Whatever the safeguards built into a clinical prevalence study of chronic illness, such as the Baltimore study, my hunch is that errors tend to occur on the side of overestimation. Doctors, after all, have been trained to find diseases. But I am here referring to a far more serious phenomenon: estimates from organizations that have a vested interest in reporting high prevalence of that disease with which they are concerned while at the same time showing that things are getting better thanks to the work of that organization.

Two examples may be given of such partisan use of data, both taken from *The Killers and the Cripplers* (National Health Education Committee, 1976). In answering the question "How has medical research paid off against tuberculosis?" the report notes that "between 1945 and 1973, the tuberculosis death rate has declined 95 percent—due in major part to the medical-research discovery of the effectiveness of streptomycin in 1945 and isoniazid in 1952" (p. 255). Knowingly or not, the authors disregard the fact that tuberculosis mortality has been declining for well over a century. In England and Wales, for example, only 14 percent of the decline in respiratory tuberculosis mortality between the mid nineteenth century and 1971 took place after the introduction of specific effective drugs (McKeown, 1976, p. 52). A dramatic-looking histogram on p. 246 of *The Killers and the Cripplers* shows an 89 percent decline in tuberculosis death rates since 1952. If, however, we superimpose the histogram on a curve showing the decline since 1900 in the

United States, we have a good illustration of how to lie with statistics while telling the truth. In 1900 the tuberculosis death rate was 200/100,000; by 1952 it had declined to 15.8/100,000, and by 1973 to 1.8/100,000. "Despite these epidemiological findings," Winkelstein (1972, p. 72) concludes, "vast and elaborate community-wide case-finding programs were extensively promoted after World War II in the United States at great cost and probably with very little effect on the established trend of the disease."

The second example that suggests the skepticism that must be exhibited toward prevalence data presented by those with vested interests is found in the estimate (National Health Education Committee, 1976, p. 186) that about 250,000 persons are suffering from multiple sclerosis; this figure gives a prevalence rate of about 120/ 100,000 persons in the United States. The cited source is one of the classic texts in the field. It so happens that I have engaged in some epidemiological work on multiple sclerosis and was surprised by this rate. My suspicion led me to check the source (McAlpine, Lumsden, and Acheson, 1972). Neither the first two chapters, devoted to epidemiology, nor the index revealed any basis for the claim. The highest prevalence rates cited for sizable populations are 60–70/ 100,000 (p. 13). A list of some forty surveys reveals only three populations with rates of over 80 (p. 6: Rochester, Minn.; Orkneys and Shetland; and southeast Norway). I am not suggesting intentional deception. I am pointing out that a vested interest shapes one's perception of the facts.

The fifth methodological issue to be considered is that of a seeming paradox. In a 1973 National Health Interview Survey, 48.7 percent of the population sample reported (or the spokesperson of the family reported) that they were in excellent health, 38.4 percent in good health, 9.4 percent in fair health, and 2.8 percent in poor health (see National Center for Health Statistics, 1976, p. 243). Even if we take into account the fact that the sample represented only the noninstitutionalized part of the population, the subjective evaluation of 87.1 percent that they were in at least good health seems to stand in sharp contradiction to the mass of data presented in this chapter. A similar report was issued over television by the Department of Health, Education and Welfare only a few days before these lines were written. The explanation is fairly simple.

Researchers generally agree that posing such broadside questions about satisfaction (about one's family, work, health) almost always elicits a widespread positive response. I am not at all saying that subjective perception of one's state of health is unimportant. As a social scientist, I would be the last to do so. My point is methodological. Research experience shows that the more an interviewer establishes rapport and goes into detailed questioning, the more the interviewer discovers elements of discontent, concern, and difficulty. Thus at one level people report that they are quite healthy; at another level they reveal substantial ailments. Both sets of data have meaning, and there is no contradiction between them.

Finally, I must take note of a possible explanation of the data that is not warranted. The claim might be made that aggregate data, such as those presented here, obscure the fact that the highest rates of morbidity are found among the elderly, the poor, blacks, and other minorities. No doubt these groups indeed have much higher rates, quite across the board, than does the rest of the population. My own work has contributed to substantiating this generalization. Nonetheless, careful examination of the data shows that higher rates for these groups do not come even close to explaining the rates of morbidity for the entire population. The salutogenic question is hardly less pertinent to white, middle-class, and non-elderly people than it is to the more discriminated-against.

Significance of Salutogenesis

I trust that I have provided some measure of evidence in support of my contention that even in the 1970s and even in the most industrialized societies, with, relative to earlier eras, high levels of standard of living, environmental control, and medical technology, a far greater proportion of the population is ill, by any conservative definition, than one might think to be the case. I anticipated that this would be true on the basis of the observation that the bugs are ubiquitous and, one might add, most sophisticated. It should, then, be clear that the mystery of health is indeed intriguing. But why is it socially and humanly important?

Let me, at the outset of my attempt to support my position that the question Why do people stay healthy? is today the crucial question, make it crystal clear that I do not contend that it should replace the older question (not that I think there is any such danger). My point is to make a plea for the allocation of a small fraction of the resources—of the funds, of the manpower, and, most important of all, of the thinking of those concerned with health and illness—now overwhelmingly, if not exclusively, devoted to the study of pathogenesis.

If, then, we can begin to understand this mystery—the mystery of survival, the mystery of why some people's health is such that they go through life for some of the time with relatively little pain and suffering—we might begin to think about applying this understanding to reduce pain and suffering among the rest of us. There is, of course, no promise that it will be within our power to do so. Conceivably, the only answer to how to stay relatively healthy is not to live—which is no answer. But if we do not attempt to even pose the question—if we remain forever in the sphere of chasing and learning to kill this or that bug or of being sophisticated and seeking general weapons that kill a number of bugs simultaneously or of avoiding "unnatural" behavior—we limit ourselves to the confines posed by the study of pathogenesis; and, as glorious as the achievements of that study have been in the past, we thereby handicap ourselves unnecessarily.

I would point to three specific reasons why the focus on pathogenesis is likely to handicap us in grappling with both the scientific problem of understanding why illness is far from deviant and the human problem of somewhat reducing pain and suffering. In each case, the salutogenic approach offers a viable alternative.

First, the pathogenic approach pressures us to focus on the disease, on the illness, on the alteration of body fluids or structures, and to disregard the sickness, in Eric Cassell's terms (1976). That is, it blinds us to the subjective interpretation of the state of affairs of the person who is ill. Some medical scientists and clinicians manage to overcome this narrow vision. Thus Cassell points to general characteristics of sickness—loss of connectedness and of feelings of omnipotence, omniscience, and control—as consequences of illness and entry into the patient role (pp. 40–44). His humanity and sensitivity bring him to the realization that these feelings also cause suffering, which the physician should try to alleviate. But even if emphasis on the disease state does not blind one to the person who has the disease, the pathogenic model binds one to an etiologic focus on the disease—that is, one limits oneself to asking, What has caused this specific disease? Even Cassell fails to ask whether the characteristics he discusses may not be of etiologic significance for disease in general. Salutogenesis, by contrast, opens up, or even compels us to examine, everything of import about people who are ill, including their subjective interpretations of their state of health.

Second, thinking in pathogenic terms is most comfortable with the "magic-bullet" approach—one disease, one cure—which explains the resistance of many to the concept of multiple causation. But even those who do not view matters simplistically find that, by concentrating on a single disease, they can seldom account for much of the variance in its development in either populations or individuals. They are, in a way, worse off than those who search for the necessary even if not sufficient cause, for eliminating necessary causes does do away with a specific disease. But in either case the assumption is that we are cleverer than the bugs and can eradicate them one by one. Rid of this illusion, we can only become pessimists. But using a salutogenic model, asking questions about what maintains health, allows us to go beyond "not smoking" or "vaccinating against polio" or "eliminating smog."

Third, pathogenesis by definition is a model that postulates a state of disease that is qualitatively and dichotomously different from a state of nondisease. The individual is sick or well. The organ is diseased or nondiseased. The condition is pathological or nonpathological. If the data presented in this chapter mean anything, they suggest that such dichotomization blinds us to a conceptualization made possible by a salutogenic model, namely, a multidimensional health-illness continuum between two poles that are useful only as heuristic devices and are never found in reality: absolute health and absolute illness. Pathogenesis asks, Why does this person enter this particular state of pathology? (or the epidemiological equivalent of this question). Salutogenesis asks, What are the factors pushing this person toward this end or toward that end of the continuum?

Chapter Two

Measuring Health
on a Continuum

Kuhn (1962) has taught us that all scientific research and the social institutions in which it is conducted and applied are characterized by a given pervasive paradigm. The dominant paradigm of Western medicine, the pathogenic orientation, has indeed produced great triumphs. Western industrialized societies have reached the most advanced stage in history in their understanding of and capacity to cope successfully with at least the physical suffering to which people are heirs.[1] Chapter One, framed within the constraints of

---

[1] This statement is not sarcastic. I am fully aware of the ills of modern societies, but the evidence points clearly to the conclusion that, by any reasonable criteria for health, Western industrialized societies have achieved the highest levels of any sizable population in history. Of course, if one wishes to prove the contrary and drags in criteria such as alienation, ugliness, and mass deceit to show how sick modern societies are, no discussion is possible.

I am also aware of the relatively recent "discovery" of the state of physical and emotional grace, almost, of the true natural person, as it were,

the pathogenic paradigm, nonetheless demonstrated that even in such societies a substantial proportion of the population manifests disease. This paradox, I suggest, cannot be explained unless we rephrase the central question and ask, Given the ubiquity of bugs, why does anyone ever stay alive and reasonably healthy? Or, to put it more formally, we cannot explain the paradox unless we adopt a salutogenic paradigm.

At the core of the pathogenic paradigm, in theory and in action, is a dichotomous classification of persons as being diseased or healthy. Our linguistic apparatus, our common sense thinking, and our daily behavior reflect this dichotomy. It is also the conceptual basis for the work of health care and disease care professionals and institutions in Western societies. Consideration of the problem of the origins of health, however, leads us to face the question of whether the dichotomous approach is adequate or whether it may not be imperative to formulate a different conceptualization of health.

This chapter, then, is devoted to an analysis of the compelling link between the pathogenic paradigm and the health-disease dichotomy and to the formulation of a continuum model compatible with and appropriate to a salutogenic paradigm. Let us look first at what goes on in the appropriately named disease care system.

Clinical Model

At any one time, people are placed, as a first approximation, in one of two categories by use of a simple, observable, and objective

---

in hunter-gatherer societies, living in harmony with the surroundings and biologically well adapted to them (see Powles, 1973, and Eyer and Sterling, 1977, who present this thesis, with a good bibliography). At present this claim derives from an ideological commitment and is hardly a hypothesis that is testable. There is certainly general agreement that my text statement is accurate with respect to the comparison of industrial and agricultural societies and that the first agricultural revolution some ten thousand years ago initiated a chain of increased food supply, brought about the aggregation of populations of substantial numbers, and saw the beginning of the predominance of infectious diseases (see McKeown, 1976, pp. 66–67). But whether Homo sapiens, in the hundreds of thousands of years before this, was healthy in a near-idyllic manner seems most doubtful. Until we have convincing evidence to the contrary, I suggest that malnutrition, violence, and accident made life quite unpleasant and short, even if not as much so as during the agricultural era.

criterion: If they have not appeared in the formal, institutionalized disease care system—if they have not become patients—they are well. If they have so appeared, they are ill. But having someone ill is distressful for personnel in the disease care system since they have never been trained to deal with ill people but rather with illnesses. The well-trained physician looks for signs that suggest a disturbance of the organs or body fluids characterized by structural alteration or biochemical change. Where data are adequate, the patient can be classified in one or multiple categories by use of the conventional rubrics of pathology, whose ultimate development is found in the International Classification of Diseases. The physician can then, one hopes, engage in treatment.

There are two residual categories. First, there is the person who shows no "objective" signs of pathology. Such a person used to be called a malingerer and was given short shrift; this is still in good part the case in those social situations, such as an army, where being classified as ill often pays off. Today, more frequently, people in this category are presumably treated more kindly; they are told that the problem is emotional or psychological. The second residual category contains those people who, having entered the disease care system and undergone a diagnostic scrutiny, have not provided adequate data for subclassification, though they clearly have something wrong. It should also be noted that the diagnosed-patient category is subdivided into those for whom nothing therapeutic can be done and those who can in some way, it is to be hoped, be helped.

Subclassification also goes on in the world outside the disease care system. Given the social costs of illness, there is great pressure in industrialized societies against entering the disease care system. (There are, of course, counter-pressures, and the pressures against entry are differentially applied. Analysis of this issue, however, would take us too far afield.) But there is some legitimate scope for "sick" people who are not patients. It is acceptable to feel bad generally or to enter a diagnostic category defined by oneself or another layperson without entering the disease care system. In such a case, the categories may bear little relationship to those in the International Classification of Diseases, and the therapies considered appropriate may be shaped by the fads of the Madison Avenue representatives of drug manufacturers or by the sociocultural group of the sick person. One finds, though, that laypersons more than professionals are tolerant of and comfortable with feeling bad in general, without lay or professional diagnostic categorization, if feeling bad is limited to relatively short, nonrepetitive time periods.

In sum, the dominant conceptual model of laypersons and practitioners alike is one that classifies people at any given point in time in the following way:

A. A nonpatient
   1. healthy
   2. sick
      a. feeling bad in general
      b. sick with a particular diagnosis of a particular "disease" as defined by oneself or another layperson
B. A patient
   1. diseased
      a. with signs sufficiently clear to allow subclassification as
         (1) a case of disease X
         (2) a case of disease Y and/or
         (n) a case of disease n
      b. with insufficient signs to allow specific disease subclassification
   2. not diseased: malingerer, crock, hypochondriac, or emotionally disturbed person.

The pathogenic paradigm leads to and is reinforced by this system of classification. It constantly presses toward the dichotomous location of people in Category Al—healthy nonpatients—or in Category Bla—a case of disease X, Y, and/or n in treatment.

For the purpose of facilitating the work of the ambulatory-care physician, this conceptualization of the health-illness phenomenon seems appropriate and useful. It is also an effective tool in the hands of the practitioner in the acute-care hospital, whose interest, concern, and responsibility are self- and socially defined as facilitating the removal of the patient from the hospital as rapidly as possible, consistent with the perceived best interests of the patient. (Unless, of course, the reimbursement system or a syndrome fascinating to the medical staff tempts one to keep the patient in treatment.)

But, more important, this conceptualization is useful for persons suffering from a constellation of painful and anxiety-arousing sensations, running the gamut from very mild to extreme, who have come to believe that the disease care institution can be of help to them.

To put the matter another way, on any given day, somewhere between 1 and 2 percent of the population of Western industrialized society (or any segment of it that has at least some services available) will be in contact with the disease care system. (The calculation is based on three components: an average of four to five ambulatory visits to the doctor per person per year, or a monthly consulting rate of 250/1,000; about 10 percent of a population being admitted to an acute-care hospital for an average stay of eight days in the course of a year; and about 0.8 percent of a population being in a chronic-disease institution at any one time. See Thacker, Green, and Salber, 1977.) Given the present level of knowledge, understanding, and technology, we have good reason to believe that the magic-bullet, diagnose-subclassify-treat approach, a concomitant of the dichotomous model, is of considerable value to those who enter the disease care system. It works, in many cases, in decreasing suffering, in avoiding complications, and, occasionally, in solving problems. And lest someone sneer at the "considerable . . . in many cases . . . occasionally" of 1 to 2 percent, let me remind the reader that we are talking about 1.5 million people a day who hurt (in the United States). The biologically oriented research establishment, which employs the same dichotomous model, and the clinical establishment, then, to my mind, are not to be dismissed. Nor, I might add, do I see the slightest evidence that any sizable segment of the population of any Western society wishes to do so. And I do not share the arrogance of some who see backwardness or false consciousness or brainwashing in their behavior.

I think that a great many serious criticisms can be leveled at the disease care systems as they exist in the Western world. But to go into this issue would require a different kind of book—which may well be more important than this book, but it is not the one I am writing. Important and fundamental deficiencies might well be remedied, changes and modifications might well be introduced that are not in conflict with the dichotomous model of health and illness we have been discussing. This model is compatible in many ways with solo practice, with Kaiser-Permanente, Group Health Insurance, the Health Insurance Plan, and other forms of group practice. It is compatible with the quasi-socialized medicine found in Israel and with the socialized medicine of Great Britain and the Soviet Union.

I am here concerned with the unfortunate consequences of the dichotomous model—consequences that will obtain as long as this model continues to hold sole sway in the training and practice of physicians and other personnel. I touch on this issue only briefly in this chapter, as a way of introducing the necessity of at least an additional, if not an alternative, paradigm. In Chapter Eight, devoted to an analysis of the health care or disease care institution in the light of the fundamental thesis of this book, I contrast the implications for this institution of alternative paradigms. There, both ideological and social-structural issues are considered in full. For the present, I would but take note briefly of the inherent implications of the dichotomous model.

Eric Cassell (1976), among others, has movingly called attention to the general psychological needs that patients bring into every encounter with the doctor. He does not preach, urging physicians to be moral and humane, but cogently argues that the "healer's art" of considering such needs is an essential part of the diagnostic and therapeutic procedure. Patients simply get better more thoroughly and more quickly or suffer somewhat less when the curer also seeks to be a healer. (For a more profound and systematic analysis of the distinction between illness and disease, see Kleinman, Eisenberg, and Good, 1978.) My colleague Shuval has raised the same issue from a sociological point of view, inquiring into the latent, "nonmedical" functions of the medical institution (Shuval, Antonovsky, and Davies, 1970).

Cassell traces the failure to meet psychological needs to "those factors in the history of medicine that, in artificially separating the person from the disease, have directed our awareness away from the nexus of the problem" and to "the failure of both physicians and society to realize that medicine is inherently a moral profession" (p. 119). But Cassell does not see that the trained incapacity to focus on anything but the specific disease at hand is intimately linked with what he himself has thoroughly internalized: the dichot-omous model. Throughout, Cassell urges physicians to see patients as persons, by which he essentially means that physicians should be concerned about the emotional as well as the organic aspects of dis-ease. But if one conceptualizes all sickness problems as disease prob-lems (as qualitatively different from a state of health), no matter how broadly one views the disease problem, I am skeptical about how one can come to see the person. This is all the more true when the technology at one's disposal provides a fascinating set of toys. The medical student, trained only in hospitals with a focus on inter-esting diseases and armed with the dichotomous model, will in-evitably continue to be concerned with the particular, organic disease.

Another consequence of the dichotomous model is the failure to ask why the patient came into the disease care system. The task of ascertaining the appropriate diagnostic category and providing appropriate therapy is either quite simple and routine and uninter-esting or complex, mysterious, troubling. In either case, the patient's history as a person is hardly seen as relevant. When diagnosis is simple, the patient's history is superfluous; when diagnosis is com-plex, there is too much else to do; the medical history in such a case is hardly adequate, to put it mildly.

A regular feature of the *New England Journal of Medicine,* "Case Records of the Massachusetts General Hospital," demon-strates this problem most depressingly. In the issue of October 13, 1977, Case 41-1977 is about a sixty-eight-year-old man. Poor? Rich? White? Black? Married? Widowed? We do learn the details of his rich disease history. After his most recent hospital spell of forty-three days, he was home for four weeks before his present ad-mission. "At home he was lethargic and anorexic." But as to what might have gone on in whatever is called home that might help to explain his present condition and be relevant to prognosis, not a word from any of the learned, outstanding clinicians.

If the model we have been discussing, which divides people into patients/diseased and nonpatients/healthy categories, is related to failure to see the patient as a person even in the social situation of present interaction with the physician and if it is related to failure to see the past of the person as relevant to that person's current and future health, then we should certainly not be surprised that it leads to the disease care institution's totally excluding nondiseased persons from consideration and denying responsibility for them. Fortunately or not, as we have seen in Chapter One, such exclusion, over a relatively short period of time, affects only a minority of the population (when there are no barriers to access). That this is the case may well be linked precisely to the dichotomous model—to the failure to allow, even in one's thinking much less institutionally, any perceived relationship between the person as a healthy nonpatient and the same person as a diseased patient. To put my thesis here within the terms of reference of this book, unless the problem of salutogenesis is confronted, confronting the problems of pathogenesis is likely to be a Sisyphean task.

Public Health Model

Thus, the disease care institution, organized around the problem of pathology, is most comfortable with the individual patient who has come down with a diagnosable disease for which effective therapy is available. What may with some legitimacy be called, by contrast, the health care institution of Western societies has a radically different cast. First and probably foremost, it is concerned with groups—whether geographically, politically, or socially defined—rather than with individuals. Second, it is concerned with control of the environment, its aim being to prevent the outbreak of diseases.

Epidemiology is one of the major scientific disciplines that have developed in the service of the health care institution. There is no doubt in my mind that the epidemiological conceptualization of the health-illness phenomenon, the model or paradigm used by epidemiologists, is powerful and, for some purposes, far more powerful than the clinical model we have been discussing.

First, epidemiologists are aware of the iceberg phenomenon. They assume, with adequate evidence, that for every case of a disease that has been brought to clinical attention—that has come within the scope of the disease care system—there are additional cases below the surface—cases not known to the "authorities."

But, second, if there is thus an inherent temptation for epi-

demiologists to find more cases, they are kept in check by methodological sophistication and compulsiveness, which are probably the
central norms of the profession. The epidemiologist is tough minded,
unable to accept a case unless clear criteria are rationally specified
and measurable. Clinicians are kept in line by conscience and by
whatever system of peer review they may be subject to, which presumably prevent mistaken diagnoses; but intuition, art, and clinical
skills are necessarily acceptable in arriving at a conclusion. After all,
one must act. The epidemiologist has the luxury of rejecting such
subjectivism.

Third, the sine qua non of the epidemiologist's professional
activity is to go beyond description and enter the field of analysis, to
deal with causation. As such, it rounds out, complements, the field
of laboratory and clinical research. But its core and strength are its
understanding of causation as based on the study of group rather
than individual differences.

The epidemiological, or public health, model, then, is quite
different from the clinical model. It is concerned with "real" numbers; it is concerned with the distributions of cases in groups; and it
is concerned with causation.

Much as I acknowledged considerable value in the conceptual model used by clinicians, I would certainly grant value (of both
a pragmatic and a scientific nature) to the public health model.
Rational planning of care-delivery systems is dependent on the information that flows from work based on this model. Further, the
model opens up the possibility, hardly available to the clinical
model, of allocating resources to prevention and early detection of
disease as supplements or alternatives to diagnosis and therapy.
(For one of the most sophisticated attempts to cope with the problems that arise for a self-maintaining health care plan (Kaiser-
Permanente)—a plan that has an explicit conceptual commitment
to a modified clinical model that allows for prevention and early
detection—see Garfield, 1970, and Garfield and others, 1976. The
fourfold classification is described in Chapter One.) Scientifically,
epidemiological study, reinforced by the concept of multiple causation, opens the way for gaining understanding of disease causation.

Having, then, given what may sound like even higher marks
to the public health model than those I assigned to the clinical

model, I must take note of the common element of the two models—
the element that I maintain is a crucial limitation: Both models are
based on a dichotomous classification of all people as healthy or
diseased. The clinician wants to diagnose and cure the patient. The
epidemiologist wants to prevent people from coming down with a
disease or, at the least, wants to identify the disease early so that
action might be taken to prevent degeneration. But the shared
focus is always on the disease. The epidemiologist, perhaps precisely
because of the compulsion for scientific classification, insists on the
dichotomy as much as does the clinician.

Why the strength and persistence of this dichotomous approach? The source, I suggest, for both clinician and epidemiologist, is the fundamental commitment to the question of pathogenesis. As long as one asks why people get sick, one must inevitably
begin to talk not about disease but about diseases or a disease. Once
again, let me make it crystal clear that in putting matters this way
I am not in the least belittling the work of clinicians and epidemiologists. The question of pathogenesis, the dichotomous model of disease and health that it requires, and the research and action that are
shaped by the question and the model are, as I have tried to spell
out, important. But they—as probably all other phenomena characterizing human existence—have their inherent contradictions; they
not only limit inquiry but militate against even seeing that there are
boundaries. What lies beyond these boundaries I now explore.

Continuum Model

I do not claim that one can arrive at a continuum model
only by posing the problem of salutogenesis. But, unless one is
brought to the "right" answers by the "right" questions and unless
one finds that these answers give one power, for theoretical or applied purposes, such answers may soon be relinquished as fads. Let
us briefly consider a number of examples of formulations of the
continuum model of health and disease. I trust that it is clear that
I have chosen these only as examples and certainly do not mean to
imply that Cochrane (1972b), Susser (1974), and Fanshel (1972)
are the only ones who have developed continuum models.

Cochrane (p. 89) reviewed "the evolution of the ideas of my

colleagues and myself in relation to the measurement of ill health."
As a medical student he had been "taught that there was a simple
dichotomy between ill and healthy people." But after collecting a
great many biological measurements from the community, he was
struck by what seemed to be the extensive distributions of "abnor-
malities." These could not be clearly separated into the clinician's
two groups of sick and well; in fact, they showed no bimodal distribution whatsoever. Nor did he find the notion of normality and
standard deviations of any use whatsoever in view of the fundamental question he posed: What should a clinician do? Unlike most
who have asked this question, Cochrane, who did not allow himself
to remain oblivious to the iceberg aspects of the data he had collected, did not reject the continuum model. Instead, he hit upon the
solution of concentrating on "finding the point(s) on the distribution curve where treatment begins to do more good than harm."

This, then, is one step forward. Cochrane and his colleagues
have rejected the ill-healthy dichotomy and have said: Let us look
at a wide variety of radiological, hematological, electrographical,
and biochemical indices; on the basis of current knowledge, which is
always changing, let us act where we have good evidence to show
that our actions do more good than harm. They seem to have substituted these indices for the more traditional disease categories.
Thus, instead of saying that the population is divided into those
who have diabetes and those who do not, they would say that the
population has a given distribution curve of blood-sugar levels and
that, given present knowledge, X seems to be the cutoff point where
treatment will do more good than harm. This for blood-sugar levels,
hemoglobin, intraocular pressure, and so forth. Cochrane grants
that the great weakness of this approach is "its limitation to uni-
variate analysis at present" (p. 92)—that is, to a total failure to
confront the problem of overall health and illness. The rejection of
the dichotomous model inculcated by medical schools and of the
disease-categorization bind marks what may be a useful guide to
clinical practice; it does not, however, open up the way to new
theoretical questions.

Quite a different conceptualization of health and illness,
legitimately identified as a continuum model, is advanced by Susser (1974) in his analysis of the place of value systems and social

structure in the "definition of health." The health care or disease care system, Susser argues (p. 541), always deals in some way with three levels of health: the organic—"organic and physiologic disorder best described as disease (if in process) or as impairment (if static and persistent)"; the functional—"a subjective state of psychologic awareness of dysfunction best described as illness (if in process) or as disability (if static and persisting)"; and the social—"a state of social dysfunction, a social role assumed by the individual, best described as sickness (if in process) or as handicap (if static and persisting)."

Susser points out, as I read him, that all three levels of health involve conceptions of normality. Normality, however, can be conceived of in three senses. "In a first sense of pathology, normality is generally perceived as dichotomous; the disease is either present or absent." In the statistical sense, "normality for a specified condition is defined from its modal distribution in a population"; such conditions include mental deficiency (see Mercer, 1972, for an excellent discussion of this issue), hypertension, and obesity. In the social sense, normality is defined by values, by notions of how things ought to be. In actuality, Susser seems to relate his discussion of normality to the organic level, but I see no reason to limit it in this way. The focus of Susser's paper is on how values and social structure shape the attention paid to each of the three levels of health and illness, the choice of the appropriate concepts of normality (and, subsequently, the breadth of social phenomena that are subsumed in the workings of the health care or disease care institution).

I have introduced this summary of Susser's paper because I think it presents one significant way of arriving at a continuum model of health and illness, even though Susser does not explicitly commit himself to this model. Both the statistical and social senses of normality, it seems to me, compel adoption of a continuum model. But Susser's paper makes a further contribution in that he takes us beyond the sole concern with the organic. "The functions of the health professions relate to each of these levels of organization of health states" (p. 542), he points out, and it behooves us to consider consciously how this relationship works.

Susser, then, has provided an expanded model in two senses. First, he views it as essential that health and illness be conceived of

in broader terms than those of the unidimensional organic-patho-
logical model. Second, at least implicitly and at least with respect to
the functional and social levels, he suggests that people are ranked
on a continuum. Also, he says that "values and social structure account for much of the lack of correspondence between the existence
of organic disease, of illness, and of the sick role" (p. 541), though
he does not attempt to develop a systematic account of the relationship among the three levels. These contributions notwithstanding,
we are left with a model that is still shaped by the pathogenic orientation, with its constant pull toward dichotomy and its concern with
the disease, the illness, and the sick role, or the impairment, the disability, and the handicap.

A good example of a third approach to the definition of
health using a continuum is found in a paper by Fanshel (1972).[2]
Explicitly committed to an operational definition useful "in making
decisions affecting the allocation of resources and the kind of research required in the health services" (p. 319), Fanshel built his
model around one variable: functioning. "A person is well if he is
able to carry on his usual daily activities. To the extent that he cannot, he is in a state of dysfunction, or deviation from well-being"
(p. 319). Fanshel has, then, committed himself to the third of
Susser's levels. Fanshel recognizes that functioning is a matter of the
social definition of appropriate activities for specific individuals.
Application of the index would require subdivision of the target
population into cohort subsets, with specification of the socially expected role behaviors for each cohort.

The index itself consists of a series of states and describes
"the extent to which anyone in a specified state is able to carry on
his usual daily activities" (p. 319). Eleven ranked states are briefly

---

[2] This is only one of the continuum models developed in recent years
that, because their concern is operational, employ mathematical tools in
constructing health indices. The Clearinghouse on Health Indices regularly
reports both publications and research projects that use continuum models.
Since my purpose here is not to review the field, I have limited myself to
considering Fanshel's paper. It is of some interest, incidentally, that Fanshel,
a professor of electrical engineering, relies on the approach developed by
one of the leading theoretical sociologists (Parsons, 1951, chap. 10).

described, ranging from well-being through dissatisfaction to isolation, coma, and death. It would not be in place here to discuss the
details of this scale; the subsequent issues raised by Fanshel relating
to prognosis, population, and duration for given states; or the at-
tempted mathematical application to the specific problem of investment of health resources in a program for control of venereal
diseases.

There is little doubt that this paper is a contribution toward
the purpose for which it is intended: to develop an operational tool
to facilitate rational decision making in the allocation of health
resources. One may be somewhat skeptical about the extent to which
the instrument is indeed valid and reliable. One may reject the
proposal that the social value judgments admittedly necessary to
apply the instrument be made by "those responsible for the . . .
[health-delivery] services, the secretaries of state and their admin-
istrators" (p. 324). But for our purpose, that of understanding
the factors that are salutogenic, the school that this paper repre-
sents cannot be of much help. Fanshel writes, "It is important to
note that no statement has been made as to the cause for lack of
well-being" (p. 320). When he develops this point a bit further, as
well as in his later application to venereal diseases, the fundamental
distinction between Fanshel's approach and my own becomes clear.
When he thinks of causes, as well as when he thinks of action, his
reference is still to concrete diseases.

Again, I do not wish to be misunderstood and thought to be
disparaging. I see the development of this continuum scale and of
others of a similar nature, which focus on the functional consequences of diseases, whatever they may be, as valuable and of major
practical significance. (See, for example, Rutstein and others, 1976,
who write: "There are no easily measured quantitative definitions
of 'bad health,' 'average health,' or 'good health.' Our proposed
system overcomes this difficulty by establishing quantitative negative
indexes of health. Cases of unnecessary disease and unnecessary disability and unnecessary untimely deaths can be counted" (p. 586).)
Such scales are major attempts to answer the clinical and epidemiological questions of pathogenesis. But posing the question this
way cannot help us explain the mystery of how people manage

somehow to keep close to or move close to the healthy end of the continuum, however defined.

WHO Definition

Before turning to a discussion of the breakdown concept, which is my tentative proposal for the appropriate conceptualization of health, I wish to consider what is probably the most famous definition of health in the second half of the twentieth century, that of the World Health Organization (WHO), as stated in the preamble to its charter: "Health is a state of complete physical, mental, and social well-being and not merely the absence of disease or infirmity."

I admit to having passed through three phases of reaction to this definition. At first, it seemed to me a most laudable formulation of one of humanity's most ardent wishes. What could be more appropriate than the statement of such a utopian goal in a world led jointly by two cultures, differing in many ways but united in a philosophy of permanent, inevitable progress in all spheres? But not only the utopian goal and the accentuation of the positive appealed to me; even more significant, the sociologist in me thought, was the explicit realization that one could not isolate the physical from the mental and social.

This reaction, however, was not long lasting. As a researcher, as favorably disposed as I was to theoretical conceptualization as a guide to empirical studies, I soon came to see that so global a definition was far removed from an operational definition of health. This second phase of benevolent neutrality toward the WHO definition as a useless but harmless statement, however, has given way to my present position, which is one of sharp opposition. As I hope I make clear in the following pages, the resemblance between the focus on positive health and the problem of salutogenesis is quite superficial. There are two fundamental elements in my opposition.

I am not particularly troubled by specification of utopian goals. But when their social function is to keep our minds on, as the old song has it, "pie in the sky," one must be skeptical. Such goals then are not just different from, more abstract than, and more general than other goals; they are contradictory to and diversionary from such alternatives. The reader of Chapter One will not be sur-

prised that at this level of generality I much prefer Dubos' definition
of health as "a modus vivendi enabling imperfect men to achieve a
rewarding and not too painful existence while they cope with an
imperfect world" (1968, p. 67). Such an approach, while grounded
in philosophical pessimism in contrast to the Panglossian optimism
of the WHO definition, provides the dynamic orientation that is
needed in the perpetual struggle that makes some improvement
possible.

But it is not only on the philosophical level that I find the
WHO definition sorely wanting. I also find it to be the quintessen-
tial expression of medical imperialism, of the assumption that everything in life falls within the jurisdiction of the health care or disease
care system and of those who control that system. To avoid misunderstanding, I should stress that I do not question the motivations
of the framers of the definition. In formulating a utopian goal, they
no doubt had the finest intentions. Moreover, the "mental" and "social" references no doubt are based on a crucial and most welcome
awareness of the impossibility of isolating biochemical and physiological elements of human existence from other elements. But motivations, intentions, and insights are not adequate. The WHO definition does not speak of physical (and perhaps even emotional)
well-being as being shaped by or as interacting with social well-
being. It declares flatly that everything people feel about their state
of well-being is part of health and hence within the province of the
health institution. From here, it is but a minuscule jump to saying
that all aspects of a person's well-being are appropriately under the
control of those who control the institution—a formulation that, as
will become quite clear in Chapters Five and Eight, is absolutely
contrary to the thesis of this book. The sense of coherence, to anticipate, is hardly strengthened by having the health institution responsible for all aspects of people's lives.

To put the point in other words that, unfortunately, have
not been left as mere words since the WHO definition became a
sacrosanct phrase: Whatever the powers that be do not like enters
the proper sphere of medicine: political dissent, whatever the social
system, has led to locking people up "for their own good"; and sex
education, family planning and abortion, divorce and homosexual-
ity, along with underachievers and overachievers, dropouts and

jocks and grinds—all these and many more fall within the province of health with the blessings of WHO. There is no inherent leftist or rightist, liberal or conservative bias to the WHO approach. The appropriate distinction is between the powerful, who can use so benevolent a definition with a clear conscience, and the powerless.

I am thus convinced that the WHO definition of health deserves severe criticism. Yet it would be quite unfair to end on this note without considering one important venture that is based explicitly on the WHO definition. Breslow (1972, pp. 347–348) presents his argument as follows: "Our concept and measurement of health has generally focused on ill health. . . . This focus on pathology in the measurement of health probably arose from the fact that for most of human existence the health problem facing society, and medicine in particular, has been overcoming disease. . . . By the mid twentieth century . . . [the health problem] no longer consisted solely, or even largely, of being threatened by early death or specific diseases. . . . The control of previously epidemic diseases and the fact that the chronic diseases developed insidiously . . . created an essentially new kind of health problem."

It seemed to Breslow and his colleagues (Belloc, Breslow, and Hochstim, 1971) in the Human Population Laboratory of Alameda County, California, that this analysis led to the WHO definition of health. They set about examining this concept of health and formulating, in quantifiable terms, a measurement of "health in the generic sense." Being committed to the "triumvirate nature of the [WHO] concept—physical, mental, and social well-being—they thought it useful to seek a single method that would permit simultaneous assessment of all three components" (Breslow, 1972, p. 350).

At this point, however, conceptual clarification seemed to give way to methodological effort, which finally led to a seven-point spectrum as a measure of physical health. The table detailing the scale is headed "based on disability, impairments, chronic conditions, symptoms, and energy level" and consists of: severe disability, less disability, two or more chronic conditions, one chronic condition, symptomatic, low to medium energy level without complaints, and high energy level. Two further scales were devised. The first is an eight-item index of mental health—for example, feelings of being depressed or on top of the world. The second, a social-health index, measures the extent to which the individual is a functioning member of the community. It incorporates employability, marital satisfaction, sociability, and community involvement.

Clearly, Breslow and his colleagues have gone a long way toward meeting the objections that the WHO definition of health is impossibly abstract, philosophically utopian and misleading, and static. They have made a most important contribution in developing and testing a usable, sensible, and scientific tool. Their theoretical bias—an orientation toward the healthy end of the spectrum—is one I share. They have, however, failed to overcome two major weaknesses. First, their index of physical health disregards its multidimensionality and reflects a professional medical bias. Second, they have blithely fallen into what I believe to be the dangerous trap of the WHO definition in devising indexes of mental and social health. I shall, toward the end of this chapter, return to this issue.

Breakdown, or Health Ease/Dis-ease, Continuum

The central thesis implicit throughout this chapter is the contention that as long as we remain in bondage to the question of pathogenesis, we will fail to see that there are two distinguishable, fundamental questions. The first seeks to explain why a given person comes down with a specific disease and another person does not come down with that disease. On the epidemiological level, the question is simply expanded to higher and lower group rates of that disease. An important offshoot of this approach is, for those concerned with action, to find an appropriate immunological or therapeutic solution for the specific disease even before it is understood or explained. For the nth time, I should stress that I do not disparage the question of pathogenesis or the health care or disease care institution that functions on its basis.

But only when we turn to the mystery of salutogenesis, when we become aware that, with all the action and all the research in the world, so many of us so much of the time have been, are, and will continue to be sick, can we begin to see that there is a radically different question. One can put this question in a number of ways. My own preference is to ask, How can it be explained that a given individual, in this miserable world of ours, has not broken down? Or, in a group version, how come this group has such a relatively low proportion of people who have broken down? Obviously, this is a first approximation of the question. But it is adequate to point up that the focus of concern is the ease/dis-ease continuum rather than the health-disease dichotomy.

To ask about a specific disease is to narrow one's search to specific, disease-relevant factors. To ask about ease and dis-ease is to ask about generalized factors that are relevant to all diseases. And to ask about health ease, that is, to seek to explain what facilitates our movement toward the most salutary end of the breakdown continuum, is to search for weapons that may be far more potent in decreasing human suffering than is any specific disease-preventing or disease-curing factor. (Theoretically, it is quite possible to derive hypotheses about generalized factors through the study of individual diseases. This can happen when one is struck, time and again, by the fact that the same factor seems to show up in disease after disease. In practice, such generalization from specifics does not seem to have happened.) I fully grant that the search for generalized factors may turn out to be totally chimerical or that if some answer or answers are discovered, there will be no way to apply them. Not to ask the question, however, would be, I profoundly believe, a sad mistake.

Sources of ideas are mysterious. Possibly my interest in generalized factors relevant to dis-ease stems from my own childhood experience that chicken soup was the appropriate preventive, curative, and rehabilitative solution to all problems. Perhaps this intuitive knowledge was reinforced much later by my becoming persuaded that tender loving care is a more sophisticated kind of chicken soup. Whatever the case may be, my serious proposal at this point is that the search is worthwhile. I do have some faith, as will become evident, that the tentative answer I propose—the sense of coherence—is in the right direction. But even if my answer turns out to be of little help, my commitment to the proposal remains.

I have now set the stage for the explicit discussion of my formulation of the dependent variable. In my first public presentation of the concept (Antonovsky, 1972), I used the term *breakdown*. I then indicated that I would have preferred to use dis-ease. But we have all been so conditioned that it is well-nigh impossible for us to read the word with a soft *s* or to assign any meaning to it other than some medical category. The term *breakdown* seems to have caught on, and I shall continue to use it, asking the reader to bear with me and to keep in mind that the fully appropriate term is *the ease/dis-ease continuum.*

Having worked closely with Louis Guttman for years, I was influenced in defining breakdown by his facet theory (Guttman, 1974). This theory enjoins one, in formulating at the conceptual level a definition that will be subsequently operationalized, to specify the facets, or dimensions, of the phenomenon one is trying to define. Facet theory is based on the assumption that social phenomena are, by and large, most adequately understood when they are seen as multidimensional. Obviously, no ironclad rule can specify which facets of a phenomenon are sufficiently significant to be chosen for inclusion in a definition. One designs a tool with care and thought and then subjects it to public test.

With all due sensitivity to dynamics and change, the definition of breakdown starts out by viewing it as a state or condition. Further, its referent is the ecosystem of the individual organism. Once a person is located, at a given point in time, in a given category on the breakdown continuum, one can consider going further to extrapolate in time and in social space. That is, one can ask about that person's location on the continuum in the past and in the future; one can get data about other persons in the family, community, social class, and so forth. But the starting point is to ask, Where is the person now?

The sources of a faceted definition—the literature (scientific and otherwise), theoretical considerations derived from other areas, such as biology and criminology, intuitive hunches and representations—are varied. It seemed to me that one could most usefully conceptualize breakdown by selecting four crucial facets: pain, functional limitation, prognostic implication, and action implication.

Pain. Pain is an extremely complex, little-understood phenomenon, and yet it is universally known as a "personal, private sensation of hurt." (See Weisenberg, 1977, for a comprehensive review. The quote is from R. A. Sternbach, cited therein, p. 1009.) Laypeople and scientists alike may be baffled in trying to define the concept precisely. None of us, however, from the time we acquire language, whatever language it may be, have any difficulty in knowing what we mean when we say "it hurts." Nor does anyone have difficulty in answering a question along the lines of "How much are you in pain?" Cultures may vary in the extent to which they have developed fine distinctions in vocabulary, but none have ignored the phenomenon. It also seems clear that the phenomenon is closely associated with some health disturbance, with a pathological process.

It is crucial, moreover, to differentiate between pain in its health-related context and a variety of negative sensations and emotions for which the same words are often used. We often feel pain, we say, when a loved one dies, when we lose a tennis match, when our candidate fails to get elected, when we are rejected. Yet sad and sorrowful as such blows may be, it would be falling prey to what I earlier called medical imperialism to include such suffering within the sphere of breakdown. My tendency, then, is to limit the use of the pain concept in this context in the following way. I am convinced that pain is an essentially subjective phenomenon and must be measured as such. Whatever the ultimate achievements in neurophysiological research, the emotional-motivational aspects of the pain phenomenon are crucial at least for behavioral, response outcome. This conviction also leads to the conclusion that one must allow the person whose breakdown status one is measuring to decide whether the pain is related to health or not. I would, then, ask: "Is there any state or condition of your health, general or specific, that you feel is painful? Do you have no painful condition, mild pain, moderate pain, severe pain?"

I am fully aware of the wide cultural and individual (and even intraindividual-situational) variation that characterizes responses to such a question when objective observation (that is, clinical examination) would lead one to expect relative homogeneity. This variation poses no difficulty; rather, it points up the importance of defining breakdown in multifaceted terms because such variation leads one to ask questions that might not be asked when one is limited to a single-faceted definition. Concretely, encountering a person who reports severe pain but no functional limitation or "medical" condition (see below), someone with a multifaceted definition is stimulated to ask questions about the "deviant" such as: What explains the "inconsistency"? Will the person's health behavior differ from that of others in the same categories of the other facets who report no pain? What is the likely breakdown prognosis (that is, can we find typical paths of movement up and down the breakdown profiles)? I believe these are extremely important clinical and research questions.

Functional Limitation. It is quite flattering to a sociologist to see how nonsociologists have become enthusiasts of role theory. The extent to which functional limitation, which more often than not is used primarily in the sense of role performance, has been seen as a core component of sickness is considerable. There is no doubt in my mind that this is not only a valid insight but that it is universally the case. That is, when people in any given culture talk about illness, they invariably imply a limited capacity to engage in appropriate role performance. This limitation may be temporary or enduring, partial or total, but when one is socially defined as sick, one is excused from fulfilling the normative functional expectations. Thus Fanshel (1972) explicitly built a health index on the basis of the extent to which one is able to carry on one's usual activities. Breslow (1972) also stresses functional limitation as a major basis for a physical-health index, while Susser (1974) uses functioning as one of his levels of health.

There are, I suggest, three major difficulties with this formulation of functional limitation. First and probably foremost, insofar as the implications for many, many persons go, there is an inherent tendency to see the functional limitation and the person as coextensive. This connection has been most perceptively analyzed by Scott in his study of people who have visual limitations of varying extents (1969, particularly pp. 22–23). He points out that we have in our society gone far beyond the fact that "the absence of vision prevents a person from relating directly to his distant physical environment" and have created an all-encompassing social category, the blind. Occupants of this category are then socialized to adhere to the special, all-encompassing norms appropriate to a member of the blind. We have similarly categorized the "functional limitation" that ranges from perfect pitch to total tone deafness. "Mental retardates" too are related to in our society, by and large, as are the blind rather than as people with varying limitations on their performance of specific activities.

The second weakness often apparent in the use of functional limitation with respect to health status is, in a sense, the obverse of the first. If the person with little vision or with low intelligence (or perhaps, in pre-Rooseveltian days, with little lower-limb mobility) is seen as coextensive with his particular limitation and cut off from functional activity that he may be quite capable of performing, one also finds the person who, though perfectly capable, technically, of performing the social roles deemed appropriate by society chooses to opt out. Thus the objective observation as to whether a person is performing the social roles one (society? Big Brother?) would expect him or her to perform places in the diseased category those who do not accept the dominant normative expectations of their society. In less benevolent eras, such people were punished or ostracized; today, they are seen as sick, and the attempt is made to heal them.

The third weakness I would note is related to the second but differs in that it focuses on the relationship between normative expectations and given objective facts. In a hypothetical society in which adults are supposed to become parents can sterility be classified as a functional limitation? As long as one accepts the dominant normative expectation as the sole criterion, the answer is yes. If, however, the criterion used is the internalized expectations of the person whose health status is being examined, then the answer can be yes or no, depending on the person's expectations.

Consideration, then, of the importance of this facet, on the one hand, and of the caveats discussed, on the other, has led me to the following operational question concerning functional limitation: "To what extent, if at all, does the state or condition of your health prevent you from carrying out the activities of living that you feel it is appropriate for you to engage in—no limitation, mild limitation, moderate limitation, severe limitation?" This approach, no doubt, poses the specific problem of self-deceptive and "unrealistic" expectations. I doubt that too many people are likely to feel severely limited because their health prevents them from climbing Mt. Everest, running a marathon race, or becoming star performers in the Metropolitan Opera. But this approach has the virtue of meeting the three objections raised above without discarding the concept of functional limitations. It might be that, in most cases, phrasing the question in the usual way (that is, not adding the phrase about appropriateness) and phrasing it as I have proposed would lead to the same response. Until this possibility is tested, we have no way of knowing, and it seems to me to be preferable to be guided, in this facet no less than in the pain facet, by an explicit subjective criterion. (I regard the issue of subjectivity as of crucial significance for the intervention implications of the breakdown approach. It will, I hope, become clear in Chapter Eight, where I discuss the relationship between people in various categories of breakdown, the sense of coherence, and health professionals, that I think that it is at least reasonable to hypothesize that movement along the breakdown continuum is closely related to who defines the situation.)

Prognostic Implication. If, up to now, I have gone beyond the bounds of conventional modern medicine, it is my explicit concern here to include within the definition of the health ease/dis-ease continuum professional, institutionalized knowledge. In doing so, however, I do not think that I am departing from my search for universally applicable facets of a definition of breakdown. In every culture, I suggest, a given set of signs and symptoms is classified as having a particular prognostic implication. The same set might well be differently classified in different cultures. A seizure has been viewed variously as a sign of beatification and blessedness, as a passing and not particularly noteworthy event, as a promise of improvement (when following administration of electroshock), and as an expression of imminent death. But any given culture tends to have a predominant health-practitioner view of the set of signs and symptoms. To ignore this facet in defining breakdown would, I believe, be erring just as badly as to continue to limit oneself to the model presented by the International Classification of Diseases.

I would suggest three axes along which, in our culture or in others, a syndrome (or, if one wills, a disease) is always classified for prognostic purposes; such classification follows the lines of the natural history of that disease as perceived by the formal health care or disease care institution of the society. To dichotomize or trichotomize each of these three axes is, of course, an oversimplification and raises problems for the reliability of the classification. In order, however, to make the tool manageable, I nonetheless think it possible to dichotomize and trichotomize without doing too much violence to data. The three axes are the severity of the condition (mild or serious); whether it is acute or chronic; and whether its natural history is viewed as essentially self-limiting, stable, or degenerative.

In order to treat such a set of data as a single facet, with a manageable number of categories that can be ordered, I think it reasonable to disregard those combinations of the data that on face value or empirically are not likely to occur. The criterion for inclusion is the extent to which a category indicates a clear and present danger to life.

In contrast to the pain and functional-limitation facets, this facet must be based on the consensual fund of knowledge available to the formal authorities in the disease care institution of the society—in Western societies, to doctors. Once the physician has arrived at a diagnostic label, using the tools available, he or she is asked: "In your professional opinion, considering the medically most serious state or condition you have observed, would you say that the person has no acute or chronic condition; a mild, acute, and self-limiting condition; a mild, chronic, and stable condition; a serious, chronic, and stable condition; a serious, chronic, and degenerative condition; or a serious, acute, and life-threatening condition?"

In the one field trial in which this classification was put to the test in a limited fashion, there was some indication that, at the very least, as a first approximation, it is useful (Antonovsky, 1973). Four physicians, following a relatively limited period of training and clarification, were asked to classify 697 middle-aged women whom they examined. The classification seemed to make sense to them, and they reported difficulty with categorizing fewer than 17 of the women. Neither reliability nor validity was examined, however, and hence the proposal must be considered as most tentative.

Action Implication. A given condition—obesity, a lump in the breast, a lower back pain, caries—or a given behavior—a tic, visions, smoking, contraception—may or may not be regarded as health-related behavior in different cultures or subcultures. Once a condition is defined as related to health, however, all cultures have norms as to the appropriate action response, including the response of inaction, even though the norms may differ widely. This observation leads me to propose that an action facet be included in the definition of the breakdown, or health ease/dis-ease, continuum. The question to be asked of the professional is as follows: "Considering all aspects of the person's health, would you say that he or she requires no particular health-related action; efforts at reduction of known risk factors; observation, supervision, or investigation by the health care system; active therapeutic intervention?"

Several comments are warranted. First, it may be claimed that a wide variety of actions—or, indeed, everything one does—is related to health. In this sense, no person would ever be classified in the first category. I have, however, intentionally phrased the other alternatives to refer explicitly to more or less agreed-on (in a given society) risk factors or conditions related to disease. Thus, the first category is residual.

Second, I have explicitly committed myself to placing the onus for categorization on health professionals rather than on the persons to be classified. I have done so on the grounds that knowledge and expertise not available to the layperson provide the only rational basis for such classification. I trust it is clear that my reference to health professionals applies to professionals within a given society. What happens when professionals from different societies observe the same phenomenon but arrive at different conclusions about action is a fascinating question. Study of such situations would teach us a great deal, but the issue would take us too far afield here. Further, I hope it is clear that my discussion here is limited to classification, which should not be confused with decision making as to action. Epidemiological studies using the breakdown classification do not require that the health professional take action. The situation of the clinician who is using the breakdown approach is somewhat different. The clinician, having classified, is greatly tempted to make the action decision. This decision making does not, however, necessarily follow. My own preference is for the clinician to make available to the person an action recommendation and its rationale and for the person involved to decide. This preference not only derives from my own value prejudices but is linked to my theory of therapeutic efficacy, as will become clear in Chapter Eight.

Finally, a word about the last category, active therapeutic intervention. In some situations in all societies knowledge is unavailable, though one wishes that something could be done. These situations are particularly frustrating in an activist society. The most dramatic example is cases of what is defined as terminal illness. In such cases, nothing can be done except to make the patient as comfortable as possible, provide dignity, and let matters take their course. Since such situations are patently more serious than those that call for no more than supervision, I would classify them in the last category.

Breakdown Profile

In sum, I have proposed a conceptual definition of the breakdown, or health ease/dis-ease, continuum as a multifaceted state or condition of the human organism. Operationally, I have suggested that at any one time a person can be described as having a particular profile—that is, a score on each of the four facets. (I trust it is clear that under the term *breakdown,* which must serve me until a better term comes along, I include the entire gamut of types on the multidimensional continuum I have presented. "Low breakdown" refers to the healthy end of the continuum.)

The mapping-sentence technique involved in facet theory makes a succinct summing up of the approach possible. The sentence is presented in Table 5. Theoretically, this multifaceted definition of breakdown provides a total of 384 possible profiles ($4 \times 4 \times 6 \times 4$). In practice, in the study of middle-aged women referred to above (Antonovsky, 1973), almost two thirds of the women were classified in fourteen profiles; almost half, in six profiles. The study sample, it should be noted, included women from five different Israeli ethnic groups, ranging from Arab village women to middle-class, urban women of European origin.

It would take us too far afield to review the data and their implications, which I discuss in the published paper. (I cannot,

Table 5. Mapping-Sentence Definition of the Health Ease/Dis-ease Continuum

A. Pain

Breakdown is any state or condition of the human organism that is felt by the individual to be

{
1. not at all
2. mildly
3. moderately
4. severely
}

painful;

B. Functional Limitation

that is felt by him/her to be

{
1. not at all
2. mildly
3. moderately
4. severely
}

limiting for the performance of life activities self-defined as appropriate;

C. Prognostic Implication

that would be defined by the professional health authorities as a

{
1. not acute or chronic
2. mild, acute, and self-limiting
3. mild, chronic, and stable
4. serious, chronic, and stable
5. serious, chronic, and degenerative
6. serious, acute, and life-threatening
}

condition;

D. Action Implication

and that would be seen by such authorities as requiring

{
1. no particular health-related action
2. efforts at reduction of known risk factors
3. observation, supervision, or investigation by the health care system
4. active therapeutic intervention
}

.

however, refrain from noting the finding that only 9 percent of the women in the study sample were classified in breakdown profile 1–1–1–1. This finding, in a study conducted in 1970, was significant in shaping my interest in salutogenesis.) My concern here has been to propose both a conceptual and an operational approach to the definition of health and illness—an approach that overcomes the variety of inadequacies I have noted in reviewing alternative approaches. I would stress that my concern derives from posing the problem in salutogenic terms.

Why do I insist on putting the problem in terms of saluto- genesis? Does it make any difference, or is it not even more con- genial (and hence presumably more acceptable) to those engaged in this area to use a concept such as general vulnerability or gen- eral susceptibility, as my colleague Syme has proposed? He writes of "compromised disease defenses and increased general suscepti- bility"; "a better understanding of factors that compromise host resistance and increase vulnerability to disease, . . . factors that influence generalized susceptibility [and] those that influence the development of specific diseases" (Syme and Berkman, 1976, p. 6; Syme and Torfs, 1978, p. 47).

In principle, I have no objection to Syme's proposal to study generalized factors that make for moving down the breakdown continuum. It is, in fact, identical with my own proposal in the original presentation of the breakdown concept, as suggested by the very use of the term. I do, however, hesitate to use generalized factors because the orientation remains clearly pathogenic. In the conclusion to Chapter One, I note three reasons why the question of pathogenesis is inadequate: it blinds us to the subjective in- terpretation of the state of affairs of the person; it pushes in the direction of the single disease and single bullet; and it postulates a dichotomous, qualitative distinction between a state of disease and a state of nondisease. In the present chapter I have developed the thesis that locating a person on the health ease/dis-ease con- tinuum (or characterizing a population according to its distribution on the continuum) poses a different problem than does reference to particular diseases and opens the way for different kinds of solutions.

My hunch is that posing the problem of generalized vulner- ability rather than salutogenesis tends to be subject to the above objections. Further, it tends to focus on the "more vulnerable," continuing to assume that they are the deviants, rather than on the real deviants—those close to the ease pole of the continuum— and rather than on the factors that facilitate moving toward this end of the continuum.

If these tendencies are indeed not found, then I certainly do not have the slightest objection to the use of *vulnerability, sus- ceptibility,* or any similar term. Similarly, I do not insist on the term *breakdown, or health ease/dis-ease, continuum.* I should like to think that my concern is substantive and not semantic.

One final important remark is in order. There would seem to be reasonable ground for charging me with disregarding the central imperative of my own salutogenic orientation. The health ease/dis-ease, or breakdown, continuum as presented here essentially seems to formulate the most desirable health category in negative terms: an absence of pain, no functional limitation, and so forth. There may be some truth to this charge.

Nonetheless, if the reader is troubled by the absence of a superhealthy, positive health category, my point has not been fully clarified. The salutogenic orientation is not concerned primarily with explaining how people reach perfect health—at best, a heuristic notion—but rather with understanding the factors involved in remaining at a given point or moving up the breakdown continuum, wherever one is located on it at a given point in time. This orientation is what makes it no less a tool for understanding the fate of patients recovering from myocardial infarction than for understanding people located toward the salutary end.

Yet it may be valuable, if we are to study really healthy people, few as they are, to have some way of identifying them beyond the 1–1–1–1 category. To this end, I would propose an additional question, to be asked after the first four questions have been answered with the first alternative in each case: "You have said that your state of health is not painful and imposes no limitations. The doctor's report gives you a clean bill of health. But these are negative things. Would you say that your state of health goes beyond this, that you feel an abundance of energy, that you are what people call a picture of perfect health?"

Well-Being

I have been careful so far in specifying that my concern is with the *health* ease/dis-ease continuum. As a behavioral science teacher of medical students, I have often found myself in a bind. On the one hand, it is crucial that they learn to see health in a broad context going far beyond the physiological level. On the other hand—as indicated in my comments above on the WHO definition of health and Breslow's approach—I have considered it of the utmost importance that a clear delineation be made between health ease/dis-ease and other realms of well-being.

In *Dynamics of Wellness*, a book devoted to health well-being by and large consonant with the salutogenic orientation, the opening paper (Sorochan, 1970, pp. 9–10) reflects what I regard as unnecessary and damaging confusion. "Health is made up of many kinds of personal well-being. . . . High-level wellness is characterized by . . . adaptability to cope with and to overcome all types of stresses in everyday living, . . . ability to give way to creative imagination, . . . feelings of being a worthy member of society, . . . feelings of responsibility for others." In other words, health includes everything that can possibly be regarded by someone, or in some culture, as desirable.

In a study conducted in Israel some years ago (Antonovsky and Arian, 1972), which was part of an international study, I investigated what may be called the concept of well-being. Health, in the more limited sense, certainly assumed an important role in this study, but it was only one of literally scores of significant concerns of people. Some people were terribly troubled about the possibility of war with the Arabs; others, about the "immoral behavior" of their children; still others, about their inability to get out of debt. But there were other people who found tranquility in religion, who very much enjoyed their work, or who enjoyed sex. The study of such social indicators has been possibly the fastest-growing field of social research in the world since the late 1960s. One report developed a conceptual model that, after considerable empirical work, reduced the inquiry to about 100 concerns of perceived life quality (Andrews and Withey, 1974; Andrews and Withey, 1976; compare Taeuber, 1978).

My point is that by defining health as coextensive with the many other dimensions of well-being, one makes the concept of health meaningless and impossible to study. It is, of course, folly to deny the interaction between health well-being and other dimensions. I deal with this issue in Chapter Seven. But the nature of this relationship is one that must be subjected to theoretical clarification and empirical investigation. Health well-being must be measured separately, whether in the way I have proposed or in some other way. Only then can we clarify the forces that shape the individual's or group's location on the health ease/dis-ease continuum.

Having defined the problem as that of salutogenesis and having clarified the meaning of health by using the breakdown concept, I can now turn to the development of the conceptual model that I believe offers the greatest promise in leading to a solution of the problem. What set of factors, we shall be asking, can help us understand location on and movement up the breakdown continuum?

Inevitably, both because I have been conditioned as well as everyone else by the question of pathogenesis and because the overwhelming part of the data available asks this question, I too shall slip into asking, Why are people located on—or why do they move down toward—the dis-ease end of the continuum? I shall seek to avoid doing so and ask the reader to join me in this effort. But for those readers who have not been persuaded that salutogenesis is a different question, I would at least insist that they understand that it is dis-ease, and not disease, that is of concern in this book. As I put it when I first advanced the breakdown concept (Antonovsky, 1972, p. 540): "Given the 'right' constellation of factors, one will 'look around' for a way to break down. There are, as it were, always additional factors in one's internal or external environment which one 'chooses' and which facilitate the expression of the breakdown in one specific disease or another." It is to the study of the "right" constellation of factors that we now turn.

Chapter Three

Stressors, Tension, and Stress

I would no more deny the pathogenic role of stressors than I would the role of the tubercle bacillus as a causative factor in clinical tuberculosis. The evidence is quite strong that, in a large number of diseases, stressors appear as statistically significant risk factors. Posing the problem of salutogenesis, however, brings one up short. When the tubercle bacillus is not present, one does not get tuberculosis. But is it the case that when stressors are absent, one stays at or moves toward a low level of breakdown? The absurdity of the suggestion is not immediately self-evident in reading the stress literature. There, discussion always focuses on the highly stressed group, suggesting that the controls have not experienced stressors. In this light, let me state the central thesis of this chapter in elementary form: Stressors are omnipresent in human existence. In response to a stressor, the organism responds with a state of tension.

This state can have pathological, neutral, or salutary consequences. Which outcome results depends on the adequacy and efficiency of tension management. Poor tension management leads to the stress syndrome and movement toward dis-ease on the continuum. Good tension management pushes one toward health ease.

In this chapter I seek to clarify the nature of stressors and place their role in salutogenesis and pathogenesis in what seems to me to be a proper perspective. The concept of tension management is the focus of attention of Chapter Four. There a variety of resistance resources come under systematic scrutiny. This attempt at systematization led me to complete the salutogenesis model with the development of the sense of coherence, the subject of Chapter Five.

What Is a Stressor?

The human organism has evolved homeostasis-maintaining and homeostasis-restoring mechanisms. These regulate body temperature, blood pressure, blood calcium, and so forth, so that we may stay alive. As Cannon (1929, 1939) demonstrated about half a century ago, these exquisite mechanisms are in constant, automatic operation, responding to the constant disturbances of homeostasis that living involves. Parallel learned mechanisms in the development of personality, the cultural, subcultural, and idiosyncratic-individual responses to the minutiae of an ever-changing environment, maintain social and psychological homeostasis. In other words, in the course of living, we constantly engage in the minor, automatic expenditures of energy required to keep ourselves on even keels. Surely this is a fascinating field of study. But it would be foolish to define the relatively slight changes in our environmental field, thousands of which occur daily, as stressors.

The view of life as a constant, dynamic cybernetic system, however, is a valuable point of departure for a discussion of the stressor concept. Without qualifying as an acceptable definition, the notion that information about change requires energy expenditure for the restoration of homeostasis suggests the crucial facets of a useful definition of a stressor. First, it implies that the initial source of the disturbance can be the external or the internal environment of the organism or both. Second, it suggests that homeostasis has been upset—that a demand has been made on the organism that, given its mode of functioning at that moment, it is not capable of meeting. An additional source of energy must be called on. Note that no assumption about pain or unpleasantness is made.

The difference between a stressor and other types of stimuli, I would suggest, is, at first sight, a matter of degree. A routine stimulus is one to which the organism can respond more or less automatically, one that poses no problem in adjustment. The feedback mechanism is part of one's routine repertoire, with energy readily available to allow its functioning. A *stressor*, however, can be defined as a demand made by the internal or external environment of an organism that upsets its homeostasis, restoration of which depends on a nonautomatic and not readily available energy-expending action. I do not know whether it will ever be possible to identify empirically at what point a routine stimulus becomes a stressor in the same way that we can identify zero degrees Celsius as the point at which water becomes ice. More likely than not, there is a transition zone. This does not mean, however, that there is not a qualitative difference between stressors and other stimuli.

Given this position, the implication would seem to be clear that whether a given phenomenon, a given experience, a given stimulus is a stressor or not depends both on the meaning of the stimulus to the person and on the repertoire of readily available, automatic homeostasis-restoring mechanisms available. This approach is not at all original. It is well-nigh identical with that taken by Lazarus and Cohen (1977), who view the problem in "transactional" terms and focus on the "mediating processes" of cognitive appraisal and coping. They state that stressors are *"demands that tax or exceed the resources of the system* or, to put it in a slightly different way, demands to which there are no readily available or automatic adaptive responses" (p. 109, emphasis in original). Similarly, my approach to the definition of a stressor is concordant with the "problem-solving model" of Scott and Howard (1970). And I do not see any significant discrepancy between my approach and that of Moss (1973), even though, in referring to Scott and Howard, he writes, "Their model, we think, should not be presented as a general integrative model" (p. 51).

There is, then, an emerging consensus with regard to the

stressor concept that, in Lazarus' term, sees it as a transactional phenomenon based on the meaning of the stimulus to the perceiver. Whatever the many disagreements and the lack of clarity in the theory of stress, on this one issue there seems to be consensus. Yet I cannot go along with the implication of this consensus, paradoxical as this position may seem. Of course events mean different things to different people and are differentially threatening because of past experience, because man is a symbolic animal, and because of differences in available repertoires. But if we return to our starting point—the problem of salutogenesis—I suggest that this understanding, true as it might be, does not matter much.

Let me be explicit about what I am saying does not matter much. I agree that there are individual or group differences in the differential perception of phenomena as stressors or as routine stimuli. But if we seek to understand different levels of breakdown, then what is common to us all (or almost all) is far more important than such differences. My argument is based on two interrelated points. First, by the very nature of the human organism at the biochemical, physical, and psychological levels and by the very nature of all human cultures, there is a wide sphere of consensus about what would be perceived as a stressor. Second, and even more crucial to my argument, is the observation that even if we do differ in labeling phenomena as stressors, the overwhelming number of human beings are, most of the time, in the throes of confronting what they define as stressors. The phenomena defined as such may differ; the extent of confrontation differs relatively little.

Are Stressors Objective or Subjective?

Let me start this discussion by granting one qualification at the outset. Some individuals unfortunately are extremely deviant. They define experiences that the rest of us tend to see as minor stressors or as routine stimuli as overpowering stressors. Taking an examination, speaking in a group, entering an elevator, being touched by another are phobias in the realm of psychopathology. My case does not at all rest on the idea of phobic stressors. (If, however, George Orwell in *1984* is correct in suggesting that each of us may well have his particular phobic interpretation of a given stimulus that Big Brother can identify, then such phobias are part of the picture.)

As a point of departure, we may note that none of us would have any hesitation in identifying certain human exigencies as stressors. I here refer to physical trauma of sufficient suddenness and massivity to destroy or decisively injure a vital organ and hence result in sudden death. Perhaps falling just short of such events are what Lazarus and Cohen identify as cataclysmic phenomena (1977, p. 91), which they define as "life events . . . affecting large numbers of people, usually outside of the control of individuals or groups, and assumed to be more or less universally stressful." They refer to natural disasters, wars, bombing, and relocation.

In part of my own research, ranging from my 1963 study of multiple sclerosis (Antonovsky and Kats, 1967) to my 1972 study of overall health (Antonovsky, 1974), my commitment was to the question "Did you encounter this experience?" rather than to the question "Did you encounter experiences that you would define as stressors?" It seems to be a reasonable assumption that almost everyone would agree in defining as stressors experiences like being in a situation where the people around one are being killed, having the head of the family unemployed for months, having one's child die, or migrating from one country to another.

In taking this approach, I was following the lead largely of Selye (1956). Since he was concerned mostly with stress, defined as a general adaptation syndrome, he seemed to define a stressor as "that which produces stress" (p. 64). Working in the laboratory, he administered stressors that were noxious agents by definition: "[One can produce the general adaptation syndrome] by injecting foreign substances (tissue extracts, Formalin). Subsequent experiments showed that one can produce essentially the same syndrome with purified hormones. . . . One can also produce it with physical agents, such as cold, heat, x rays, or mechanical trauma; one can produce it with hemorrhage, pain, or forced muscular exercise; indeed, I could find no noxious agent that did not elicit the syndrome" (pp. 29–30). Note that Selye is not defining stressor in circular terms. He assumes broad consensus among laboratory workers that certain things are noxious agents. In precisely the same way, I contended that there is indeed broad cultural, if not universal, consensus that certain experiences are noxious or are stressors.

This objective, consensual approach to stressors at first seemed to be accepted by Harold Wolff and his colleagues at the Human Ecology Study Program at Cornell. Study of thousands of patients in the late 1940s and early 1950s led them to the conclusion that certain types of life events were empirically observed to cluster at the time of disease onset (Wolf and Goodell, 1968). Holmes, one of Wolff's colleagues, working with Rahe, later systematized these events in a rating scale (Holmes and Rahe, 1967). The events included in the scale, whether ordinary or extraordinary, socially desirable or undesirable, had one common theme: Each was one "whose advent either is indicative of, or requires, a significant change in the ongoing life pattern of the individual" and as such "evoked, or was associated with, some adaptive or coping behavior" (Holmes and Masuda, 1974, p. 46). In subsequent studies conducted in a variety of countries, Holmes and his colleagues found that the forty-three items in their Social Readjustment Rating Scale were given much the same rank order in weighting by many different populations. Using this scale, they assign people Life Change Unit (LCU) scores, which have been used in many studies and have been shown to be correlated with vulnerability to illness. Holmes, then, seems to be arguing that at least these forty-three life events are, objectively and universally, stressors, though of different magnitudes.

Holmes' colleague Rahe, however, suggests a departure from this view and opts for what I earlier called an emerging consensus. In his view, "In dealing with large samples one can use these mean LCU values. . . . In dealing with small groups of subjects, however, individual variation in LCU scaling may assume some importance" (1974, pp. 76–77). Rahe then proposes a Subjective Life Change Unit scaling system, in which each individual assigns a score to those of the forty-three life change events he experienced— the score representing "the amount of adjustment you needed to handle the event." Conceptually, Rahe describes this technique as "the past experience filter" (Rahe, 1974). (For a succinct review of the life-events school, see Rahe, 1978.) Wolf and Goodell (1968), colleagues of Wolff, explicitly commit themselves to this subjective approach: "Illness often occurs when an individual perceives his life situation as peculiarly threatening to him, even though his life situation may not appear to be threatening to an outside observer" (p. 206).

Hinkle, Wolff's co-organizer of the Human Ecology Study Program at Cornell, from which so many of the important stress studies have come, is likewise committed to the meaning of an experience as a potential stressor: "From a physiological point of view a man may be expected to react to the 'meaning' of information he obtains from his social environment and not necessarily to the 'objective' features of it that are discernible by others" (Hinkle, 1974, p. 10).

At the same time, one can detect some ambivalence among these scientists. Wolf and Goodell, in a lengthy and detailed discussion, write, "Important as are the upheavals of rapid social change and the cruel circumstances imposed on man by his fellows, the ordinary vicissitudes of daily life offer their share of challenge as has been pointed out. It may indeed be stated that man is always under stress of one sort or another." They then go on, in a lengthy discussion, to detail what American life is like in the twentieth century from this perspective, making the assumption that all the things they point to are stressors and are interpreted as such by all those who experience them (pp. 212–221). Hinkle too comfortably slips into phrases like "major social deprivations and demands and . . . major changes in . . . interpersonal relations" (p. 24).

In other words, though many investigators seem to pay lip service to the importance of conceptualizing stressors as subjectively experienced and interpreted, "meaningful" phenomena, in the last analysis they are aware, implicitly or explicitly, that most people viewed a fairly wide range of experiences as stressors.

Ubiquity of Stressors

It is, however, most important to take this discussion one step forward. Conceivably, there could be a large measure of agreement among people that certain experiences or phenomena are stressors. Yet at the same time they might well differ considerably in the extent to which they personally experience such stressors. Thus, in my own studies, I found considerable variation, with respondents having very low to very high stressor scores. Similarly, all the studies using the life-events scale have reported great variation. And from common observation and daily living, all of us can point to people to whom everything seems to happen and to others who seem to walk between the raindrops. In fact, two of my publications would suggest that I am at least as aware as other investigators of the substantial differences among individuals and groups with regard to their exposure to stressors. I cannot pretend that the concentration camp survivors I studied lived through no more stressors than did the control group (Antonovsky and others, 1971). Nor would I claim that poor people suffer fewer stressors than do the nonpoor (Kosa, Antonovsky, and Zola, 1969).

My thesis, rather, is that all of us throughout life, in even the most benign and sheltered of environments, are fairly continuously exposed to what we define as stressors. The range of human experience in exposure to stressors is not from very low to very high. It is, rather, from fairly serious and lifelong—in, shall we say, the typical experience of many, though far from all, comfortable middle-class readers of this book—to the unbelievable hell on earth of so large a part of the world's population. We are able to get low scorers on stressor experience because we do not ask the right questions or do not ask patiently enough and not because there really are any low scorers. But then why on earth should we expect otherwise? If in the last 150 years well over sixty million human beings have died as a result of human violence alone, how have the rest of us lived? Let us thus turn to a somewhat systematic analysis of the stressors that confront human beings.

It is, perhaps, most appropriate to start with cautious and tentative reference to two exciting fields that are largely alien to social scientists, genetics and physics. While I would not even begin to pretend to anything but the most superficial acquaintance with the ideas I shall touch on, their importance is so considerable in the present context that I have gone out on a limb. The concepts of entropy and of genetic mutation are, at the physical and biochemical level, most pertinent to the thesis that stressors are ubiquitous in human existence.

The Second Law of Thermodynamics states that the entropy—roughly, a measure of disorder—of a closed system will always increase. Maximum entropy is reached when a permanent state of no observable pattern of events in the system occurs. The total entropy of a system must increase or at least remain constant. But the law applies only to a closed or isolated system. Clearly, the human organism is not a closed system. As Schrödinger puts it (1968, p. 145): "Thus a living organism continually increases its entropy—or, as you may say, produces positive entropy—and thus tends to approach the dangerous state of maximum entropy, which is death. It can only keep aloof from it, i.e., alive, by continually drawing from its environment negative entropy. . . . Thus the device by which an organism maintains itself stationary at a fairly high level of orderliness (= fairly low level of entropy) really consists in continually sucking orderliness from its environment."

The concept of negative entropy is referred to again in Chapter Four. For the time being, our concern is with a consideration of the possibility that open and closed systems differ only in that closed systems cannot be saved by negative entropy, by sustenance or information. (See Buckley, 1968, pp. 143–169, for discussions of the links between the concept of entropy and information theory.) Thus there must be inexorable, unavoidable, immanent factors that produce entropy; in our terms, these factors are called stressors. We may find, I believe, some hint of what these factors are if we turn to genetics.

In brief, there is a genetically programmed, built-in, and ultimately victorious pressure toward senescence and death of the organism. Burnet (1974 and 1971, especially pp. 154ff.) posits two evolutionary requirements for the individuals of any species: survival to a reproductive age and death when survival no longer offers any advantage for reproduction. He particularly focuses on "abnormal mutant cells which by developing toward malignancy threaten survival" (p. 131). (In Chapter Four, Burnet's concept of immunological surveillance is considered in the context of our consideration of resistance resources.) The suggestion is that, whether through mutation of cells or other senescent pressures, the organism is constantly assailed by the stressors, the challenges, that push toward entropy.

While Burnet's interest is largely in genetically determined stressors, he by no means ignores the microbiological and other stressors of the external environment. These certainly are not to be disregarded in an age that has become conscious of environmental pollution, radiation hazards, and the like. But Dubos, too, in his text on infectious diseases (1965, p. 35), argues that endogenic microorganisms are, at least in modern societies, the major category of biological stressors: "In the classic infections of exogenous origin, the determining etiologic event of the disease is exposure to the infective microorganism. In endogenous microbial disease, the immediate cause is the environmental factor which upsets the biologic equilibrium that normally exists between the host and the microbial agents. . . . The methods . . . of the past will not prove to be effective in the control of the disease states caused by microbial agents which are ubiquitous in our communities in the form of dormant infections."

Technically, Dubos' focus on the innumerable, omnipresent endogenic microorganisms, which maintain a symbiotic relationship with the host, is best referred to as a concern with potential stressors. The latent or dormant infections of which he writes become pathogenic only under certain conditions. We now understand that these conditions are not only physical, chemical, and biological but also psychosocial. Dubos' analysis, then, is most consistent with the present thesis of the ubiquity of stressors; it presses us to view the environment as made up of inextricably interwoven strands. And it also poses, to anticipate, what will be the key question of Chapter Four: How are potential stressors prevented from becoming pathogenic?

My concern here has not been to make any pretense of expertise in the physical or biological sciences but only to indicate that they cannot be ignored in a systematic consideration of the ubiquity of stressors in human existence. I simply wish to avoid the mistake of disregarding literal bugs in a discussion focusing on figurative bugs. Let us, however, now turn to the latter, to what generally has come to be called psychosocial stressors. Today the literature is overwhelming. At the time Hinkle and Wolff were developing their laboratory at Cornell, however, the link between psychosocial stressors and health was hardly the concern of many. Thus, I find it of interest to note that the central theme of this chapter—the ubiquity of stressors—was caught in an image that appears in what I regard as a landmark book of the early 1950s, *Beyond the Germ Theory*. In it, the editor writes (Galdston, 1954, p. 13): "Viewed thus, dynamic homeostasis can be likened to a man walking a tight-rope from one end to the other, balancing himself even while he changes clothes and takes on and discards a variety of other objects." Let us consider the tightrope image systematically.

Reviewing the sources of stress, Lazarus and Cohen (1977) consider three major types. The first two differ in the number of people involved. Cataclysmic phenomena, such as natural disasters, bombings, internment, and relocation, are experiences shared by whole population groups. Events of the second type, including bereavement, terminal illness, and being laid off from work, also have the same powerful and sudden impact on the persons involved, but these typically happen to fewer persons or to a single individual. Both these types of stressors occur, Lazarus and Cohen imply, with relative infrequency—or, if frequent, only to special segments of the population. My hunch is, as I suggest below, that the data would indicate that such events are far more frequent than one might think. But it is when we turn to their third type of stressor—daily hassles—that we come close to an examination of the ubiquity of stressors. But the Lazarus-Cohen account, while extensive, is hardly systematic.

Let me attempt a systematic account of psychosocial sources of stress here. In the 1930s an international "progressive" writers' congress was held in Paris. The tone for days had been apocalyptic; speaker after speaker portrayed the imminent solution of all human problems in the paradise abuilding in the Soviet Union. André Malraux, leftist but iconoclastic, rose and, in a few words, damp-ened the euphoria: "And what of the child," he asked, "who, even in the perfect socialist society, is crushed under the wheels of a tram?" My point is simple. In all human societies, whatever the precautions taken, harsh accident is immanent. My concern here is not with the victim of the accident but with the survivor who has loved the victim and, in many cases, with the bearer of responsibility for the accident. The victim has suffered a direct physical trauma; the survivor is confronted with a psychosocial stressor. Given the rates of accidental injury and death and the rate of homicide and the fact that for each victim there are most often at least three or four persons intimately involved with the tragedy, such accidents can hardly be considered an unusual source of stressors. They are not omnipresent, except as potential stressors. But their frequency, particularly among certain groups (spouses of people who drive daily, parents of children who play in the streets, workmates of those exposed to industrial accidents), leads me to see them as a constant threat in our lives.

Consideration of accidents leads us to take a further step. By and large, stress studies focus on "What has happened to you?" Of the forty-three events on the Holmes-Rahe scale of life events, which is typical of or even better than most scales, five refer explicitly to other persons; several refer to interpersonal events. But one other, the global "major change in the health or behavior of a family member," is presumed to cover the many things that happen to those close to us. Because we are embedded in networks of social relationships, our own experiences are compounded by those of the persons with whose lives our own are intertwined. (For those many persons not so embedded, this source of stressor is not significant; the price paid for not having such headaches, however, may well be far more severe.)

I would continue this list of sources of stress by discussing an area that has become oddly neglected. As a sociologist, I am pleased by the increasing attention paid in the stress literature to social disorganization, poverty, the workplace, and so forth. Yet it seems to me that this rebellion against psychoanalysis has gone too far. It behooves us to recall that serious demands and conflicts can be rooted in the internal no less than in the external environment. The very phrase *life events,* when it monopolizes discussion, signifies a displacement from any concern with internal events (as stressors and not as reactions). The things that happen to us have become the concern of investigators. Freud himself characterized the horrors of the human condition (quoted in Schur, 1972, p. 398): "The terrors of nature, . . . the cruelty of Fate, particularly as it is shown in death, . . . the sufferings and privations which a civilized life . . . has imposed, . . . the perplexity and helplessness of the human race, . . . the suffering which men inflict on one another." Thus Freud in 1927, before Hitler, before the Gulag Archipelago, before Leningrad and Coventry and Lidice and Rotterdam, before Auschwitz, before Hiroshima. But one must go much further with Freud, into the soul of the human individual, beyond the exposure to the horrors of history. Whether drives are viewed as instinctual and biologically determined or as socially learned; whether one accepts a narrow or broad interpretation of libido; whether one is committed to viewing personality formation as an intrapsychic or interpersonal process, a book that is closed in early years or one that is rewritten throughout life—whatever the disputes about Freudian theory—it is the utmost of naivete to disregard the permanent state of underlying conflict that characterizes our inner emotional environment. The impermissible impulses are there; the ambivalence is there; the fears and anxieties, if not of mutilation then of abandonment and death, are there; the guilt and shame are there. Individuals differ (as do cultures), I suggest, not so much in the extent to which underlying emotional conflict is found. These stressors are immanent. We differ, rather, in the extent to which we can contain, cope with, and perhaps even exploit (or, as Freud would have it, sublimate) these conflicts. But the stressors are there.

Again, one need not be committed to all the ideas of the recent trend in zoology, ethology, and sociobiology to take these ideas seriously in the present context. Thus L. Tiger and R. Fox (as quoted in Becker, 1972, p. 40) see human behavior as shaped by a biogram shared by all hunting primates, involving a basic appetitive predisposition that orients them "in the direction of the search for power and self-perpetuation within a hierarchy of dominance and subordination characterized by competitiveness, the real hunger for triumph, and the celebration of triumph." Whatever the adequacy or inadequacy of this approach as an explanation of violence, evil, aggression in human existence, I would suggest that there is in us all at the least an elemental fear of being the victim of evil. At some level, we all fear being the victim of aggression, mutilation, and destruction by others. Biograms may indicate no more than potential for, predisposition to, or orientation toward certain actions; ontogeny no less than phylogeny provides us with more than enough experience to make the fear an integral, if subdued, part of our everyday psyche.

Clearly, then, there are grounds for maintaining that the

human organism is subject to constant psychosocial stressors by the very fact of having been born and survived. But we also live in ongoing social environments. I would consider these at three different levels of distance from the individual: the historical-universal, the contextual, and the immediate. It may well be that before the twentieth century what happened on a historical scale could not be considered as a significant stressor unless one were directly swept up in its wake. But today the leaps and bounds of the imagination are facilitated by the mass media. More and more of us know that a small war in one part of the world may engulf us all. We see the fighting on our screens. We can visit Verdun.

Sometimes it would seem that our own lives are fairly stable but that the immediate world around us is in the process of transformation. We cannot avoid relating to it but it is not the world to which we have learned to relate. A good case in point is a study of rural residents in North Carolina; the comparison of interest was between those who lived in counties undergoing differential rates of urbanization (Tyroler and Cassel, 1964). Their concern is with people whose own activities did not change much, but the demographic, economic, and technological contexts in which these activities were carried out changed radically. (For a broader, popular discussion of the world around us in upheaval, see Toffler, 1970.) Our assumption tends to be that such transformation is a peculiar characteristic of our modern world. That this is hardly the case is suggested by the following quote. In 1882, preparing the introduction to a new edition of a work that had first appeared in 1858, Oliver Wendell Holmes (1884, p. iv) wrote:

> This book was written for a generation which knew nothing or next to nothing of war and hardly dreamed of it; which felt as if invention must have exhausted itself in the miracles it had already wrought. Today, in a small seaside village of a few hundred inhabitants, I see the graveyard fluttering with little flags that mark the soldiers' graves; we read, by the light the rocks of Pennsylvania have furnished for us, all that is most important in the morning papers of the civilized world; the lightning, so swift to run our errands, stands shining over us, white and steady as the moonbeams,

burning, but unconsumed; we talk with people in the neighboring cities as if they were at our elbow; and as our equipages flash along the highway, the silent bicycle glides by us and disappears in the distance. All these since 1857, and how much more than these changes in our everyday conditions! I can say without offense today that which called out the most angry feelings and the hardest language twenty-five years ago. I may doubt everything today if I will only do it civilly.

But if history and the more immediate world around us supply us with a considerable panorama of stressors, I suggest, without in the least ignoring this panorama, that the daily social structures in which we are all embedded are inevitably and perpetually stressful. I would, moreover, remind the reader that my concern is with stressors as defined earlier, and not with stimuli that may upset homeostasis but for which we have readily available restorative mechanisms. This is true throughout the life cycle.

For many years, the field of child psychology preempted the attention of scientists concerned with development. Infancy and childhood, in the wake of the Freudian revolution, were viewed as replete with inherent developmental crises. Adolescence, with less study, was viewed as an age of turmoil by definition, with only occasional checks and correctives introduced by the anthropological perspective. Reaching adulthood, however, meant achieving maturity, stability, and more or less smooth sailing. With the change in demographic structure and the increasing proportion of the elderly, gerontology was launched as an important field of inquiry. The stressors of retirement, dependence, poor health, and imminent death came to be investigated. However, only in recent years has the field of developmental psychology emerged as an area that is based on the paradigm of a total normal life cycle at the core of which lies an endless series of challenges. True, sociologists had long studied particular stressors of work, family life, migration. But there had not emerged from this work a developmental view of conflict or, in our terms, of stressors over the entire life span.

To take an example. When our team first began a study of ethnic differences in adaptation to menopause, we found two overwhelming interests reflected in the literature. First, the particular concern was with involutional psychosis, a pattern that at most affected a small fragment of the population (truly, the medical-model concern). Second, the assumption was that the cessation of menstruation was invariably and almost solely the key stressor on both the hormonal and psychosocial levels. With the exception of Bernice Neugarten's team at the University of Chicago, which did a series of studies on aging, no one seemed to be aware that many other stressors were endogenic at this stage of the life cycle: for example, the empty nest, the change in social status, illness, and the possible death of one's spouse (Maoz and others, 1970). Or to take another example. One of the better collections of readings on human development, edited by one of the leading psychologists in the United States, is concerned with *"ecological validity*—the study of the developing person in the contexts in which he lives." Yet its 678 pages contain not a single word about "the developing person" beyond adolescents and college students (Bronfenbrenner, 1972).

Only with the appearance of Erikson's familiar eight-stage diagram of phase-specific psychosocial crises (Erikson, 1950) did we gain a theoretical model that is useful for studying the prototypical stressors characteristic of all stages of the normal life cycle. For present purposes, it matters little that Erikson himself has made his most brilliant and important contributions to the study of the adolescent identity crisis; it matters little whether there is adequate evidence that the prototypical adulthood "generativity vs. self-absorption" crisis is cross-cultural and universal. (Certainly Erikson is supremely aware of the historical-cultural context of psychosocial crises; see Erikson, 1968, pp. 61–65.) What matters is that he has called our attention to and given us a possible framework for analysis of the psychosocial stressors that are inherent in human existence over the whole life span.

It is manifestly beyond my ability and would serve little purpose to attempt to consider in detail these inherent stressors. Readers can fill in the details for themselves and for those whose biographies they know well. Such details, it should be remembered, are limited largely to those stressors of which we are aware; others have been banished from the forefront of our consciousness and memory. Many a mother or father can only smile in recollection of the first time they bathed their first child; many a teacher smiles

recalling his first lecture; many a spouse, sexually fulfilling and fulfilled, forgets the period of early intercourse. Both those who fail
to overcome and those who do overcome stressors have good reason
to forget the terrors of such encounters. But they were there. My
intention, rather, is to suggest a number of theoretical issues in
thinking of the inherent stressors that accompany us throughout the
life cycle. These issues are, I believe, relevant to all our social roles
and to all our personal encounters. (A detailed consideration of
stressors in the life cycle is given in Academic Press' Life-Span
Developmental Psychology series and particularly in Datan and
Ginsberg, 1975.)

The first point to be made is implicit in the above discussion.
In the most benign and stable of worlds—a world certainly no
reader of this book will ever encounter—we constantly enter new
roles, new stages, new contexts. All of these pose challenges, make
demands—that is, they are precisely what we have called stressors.
Such new entries are numerous. I know of no one who has counted
such entries (which always, it should be remembered, also involve
exits and detachments) for any population. The Holmes and Rahe
Social Readjustment Rating Scale is but a bare start in this direction, given its closed-end character and time-limited focus.

Second, we should note that anticipatory socialization is
inevitably inadequate. In training, we always know that we are, as
it were, playing a game, serious as it may be. The responsibility
and the authority are still not ours. One can always say "fingers"
(in the language of my New York City childhood) to stop the
game. Simulation has been brilliantly developed as a didactic tool,
but it is not the real thing. When we do enter a new situation, the
stressor is always considerable. We do differ on how adequately we
have been prepared to cope with it, but the most adequate socialization does not guarantee that the stressor will not be perceived as
real. Further, we may have been well prepared to fight the last war;
but the new war is inevitably somewhat different.

The third issue is raised tentatively because it requires a
fundamental assumption about human nature. I discuss it here
briefly and shall return to its consideration subsequently. Let us call
it the problem of underload. We tend to think of the stressor concept, by its very definition, as referring to overload. Yet this is not
necessarily the case. There is good reason to think that an environ-

ment that makes no demands on us, that does not confront us with stressors, is, by that very fact, a stressor. The concept of underload postulates an inherent need for sensory stimulation of moderate magnitude and complexity. This postulate can call on evidence from a number of sources. It can be linked to the considerable work on infant development, which relates comfort and sustenance to stimulation. A wide variety of studies on sensory deprivation in animals and in adults, as well as in children, point to the patholog- ical consequences of underload. Psychophysiological research points to the requirement of the central nervous system for arousal in order to function adequately. Whatever the basis for the argument, it seems reasonable to suggest that environments that do not pose challenges for one are inherently stressful. (For reference to some of the literature, see Bronfenbrenner, 1972, pp. 256–301; Frank- enhaueser and Gardell, 1976; and Wohlwill, 1971.)

Up to this point I have taken pains to emphasize the in- herent stressors that all humans confront by virtue of being human and social beings. I have argued that whatever our social, cultural, and historical locations, life is, to reiterate Galdston's phrase, a walk on a tightrope with constant changes of clothes and taking on and discarding of objects. The most elementary acquaintance with history, with anthropology, and, above all, with literature—be it the Bible, the Greeks, Shakespeare, Dante, or Dostoevsky—reveals the rarity of tranquility in human existence. The content of the dis- turbances varies in time and place. The magnitude, at most, varies from that of Watergate to that of Vietnam.

But I would here focus not on what I earlier called cat- aclysmic events. As important as they are, they are different from the internal conflicts of everyday existence that are anchored in the social and cultural organization of every society. Lazarus and Cohen are profoundly though unintentionally misleading when they speak of these as daily hassles. True, they do refer, under this heading, to the stable, chronic, and repetitive hassles of poverty. But their necessarily brief summation and citation of the literature are hap- hazard. Different environments, they are saying, can be stressful. I would suggest two fundamental reasons why all social environ- ments are inherently stressful.

One need not be a Marxist to see, permitting myself some license, the history of all social institutions as one of struggle; husband and wife, parent and child, supervisor and subordinate, priest and parishioner, doctor and patient, teacher and student, officer and soldier, representative and voter, leader and rank and file—all without exception relate to each other in a context of scarcity of resources, of power, of different perspectives and interests and motivations. To deny love, mutual aid and support, cooperation, complementarity, altruism—all that Nisbet (1973), in his survey of Western thought and civilization, calls community—is to profoundly distort. But to blind oneself to the constant, inherent conflict in all social relations, group and individual, is no less a distortion. (The sociologist reader will recognize my indebtedness to Simmel, 1955, and to Dahrendorf, 1966. For a popularized account of the intrinsic stressors in American middle-class life, see Sheehy, 1974.)

The second reason for anticipating that all social environments will be stressful derives from Merton's classic analysis (1957) of the gap between culturally inculcated goals and socially structured and legitimated means for goal achievement. Merton was particularly concerned to understand the structural origins of deviance, which he defines as rejection of means or goals or both. Because he wrote his analysis originally in 1936, it is not surprising that Merton takes as his prime example the American culturally prescribed goal of the acquisition of material goods and, certainly at that time, the socially structured impossibility, for most Americans, of achieving the goal that they had presumably internalized.

Not all human societies base role placement primarily on achievement rather than on ascription. But all societies have at least some room for mobility, if only for a few individuals. Further, all societies prize particular characteristics: beauty, skill, strength, character, virtue, whatever the particular interpretation given. Most important, all societies have scarce resources and rewards, material and nonmaterial. Even in the most rigid caste society, with the most perfect indoctrination so that everyone knows one's place, the lowliest of the low have goals that are, in theory, accepted by all as legitimate. Yet no society in history has managed to avoid structural limitations or, to put it positively, has managed to provide structured access to the goals that it has propagated.

In this context, of particular interest is a paper that seeks to bring Merton's paper up to date (Simon and Gagnon, 1976).

Merton focused on the "fetishism of commodities" unavailable to most Depression-era Americans. Merton's paradigm of different types of anomic response to the means-goal gap (innovation, conformity, retreatism, and rebellion) seemed to be adequate to account for the major behavior patterns of that time. Simon and Gagnon, however, raise the question of "the anomie potentially generated by unanticipated affluence." In essence, they ask, what happens when people do succeed in the goal achievement posited by Merton? Many, though far from all, Americans are affluent, and they are not particularly happy. The authors' expanded paradigm of responses to this situation, though fascinating, does not concern us here. What does concern us is the thesis that all societies are characterized by the dilemma of the goal-means gap in two senses. First, socially structured means for goal achievement are available to only a few in any society. And, second, would it be going too far to suggest that ultimate wisdom lies in Solomon's "Vanity of vanities, all is vanity" and that such wisdom is not reached only in old age?

Throughout this chapter I have emphasized the immanent character of the stressors in human existence. Both as an Israeli and as a sociologist, I am fully aware of the differential distribution of stressors, from historic period to historic period, from culture to culture, from group to group within a society, and from the unique life of one individual to that of another. Much of my own research career has been devoted to precisely this issue, ranging from early studies of ethnic relations, immigrant adjustment, and discrimination to work on ethnic differences in adaptation to menopause, concentration camp survivors, and social-class differences in morbidity and mortality. Vietnam is not Israel is not Sweden, poor is not rich, black is not white, and male is not female. However, precisely because the overwhelming attention in stress research has been on group or individual differences in exposure to stressors, I have insisted that even the most fortunate of people and groups know life as stressful to a considerable degree.

I have in this section pursued the thesis that stressors are ubiquitous in human existence, and I have noted eleven sources of psychosocial stressors. Since I have not used subheadings, it may be useful to list these: accidents and the survivors; the untoward experiences of others in our social networks; the horrors of history in which we are involved; intrapsychic, unconscious conflicts and anxieties; the fear of aggression, mutilation, and destruction; the events of history brought into our living rooms; the changes of the narrower world in which we live; phase-specific psychosocial crises; other normative life crises—role entries and exits, inadequate socialization, underload and overload; the inherent conflicts in all social relations; and the gap between culturally inculcated goals and socially structured means.

I have set this list of stressors inherent in the human condition against the background of the potential stressors posed by genetic and microbiological factors. My concern here has not been to engage in a stringently systematic analysis of psychosocial stressors. Some readers may find inadequate differentiation between one source and another (accidents are part of the untoward experiences of others). Others may be troubled by unproven assumptions (underload as a stressor) or by inadequate consideration of certain types of stressors. Most important, I have by and large disregarded the historical and sociocultural contexts of stressors. I have done so intentionally, not because I am unaware of how such contexts shape and determine the particular expressions of stressors but because my concern has been to suggest that in all societies, under all historical circumstances, psychosocial stressors are inherent in human existence.

I have presented this thesis orally before various audiences (true, all with university affiliations, but such audiences probably only accept the thesis with more difficulty). I have asked them, as I would ask the reader, to test the thesis in the light of their own lives. I have yet to find anyone who has not known tragedy, sorrow, challenge, disruption, and conflict as steadfast accompaniments of living.

Let me make my position completely clear. I am fully aware of the joys and pleasures, the ecstasies and simple satisfactions, and the sense of achievement, of happiness, and of creation that men and women and children find in life. I could have, though possibly with not quite equal cogency, written a paean to history and the life of the species. One part of the picture need not blind us to the other. But, it will be recalled, the problem I set out to investigate was that of salutogenesis. One possible explanation of how people move toward the ease pole of the breakdown continuum was that they are subject to a low level of stressors. I trust that the inadequacy of this explanation is now obvious. I believe there is ample evidence for rejecting the significance of the transactional conceptualization of stressors, which emphasizes the importance of perception and of appraisal. We all walk a tightrope and are fully aware of it.

The data of Chapter One perhaps now begin to become comprehensible. But then the mystery thickens: How do any of us manage and even manage well? Before we begin to deal with this question, one further issue must be discussed, if only briefly.

Stressors on the Group Level

Thus far I have discussed stressors as experiences that individuals confront. The individual has remained the focus of attention even when the same phenomenon is perceived by many individuals as a stressor and has an impact on the lives of many members of a group; this is the traditional epidemiological approach, which deals with the proportion of individuals in a given population who experience X, in this case, a stressor. But it is no less important to examine the possibility of applying the same approach at the group level. To what extent, we now ask, can we describe social groups—communities, nations, social classes, racial and ethnic groups—as characterized by stressors? Or, to put it a bit more elegantly, as living in stressful situations? It is important that the meaning be clear, for the same issue will emerge again when we deal with the resistance resources available to, and the sense of coherence of, a social group. I am referring to the objective, sociological situation of the group. How individual members of the group perceive and react to the situation is a different question (see Durkheim [1897], 1951).

The most extreme proponent of what is known in sociology as consensus theory would grant that no social group is ever so integrated, cohesive, and consensual that it knows no conflicts or stressors. Nor would that person deny that human history has known few groups so isolated and living in so benign an environment that stressors from the external environment are unknown. The most extreme conflict theorist would agree with the consensus theorist that no group can last long when it is perpetually bombarded by the stressors of internal conflict and attack from without.

What differentiates the two schools of thought is not so much the extent to which a social group is stressor ridden. This is a matter of empirical investigation (though it is true that, armed with one model, one tends to find consensus; armed with another model, one finds conflict). The crucial difference between the two in viewing the stressors that do exist in any social group is in seeing them as primarily exogenic or endogenic. Consensus theorists tend to see stressors that come from outside the group as accidental and not inherent in the nature of the relationship of the group to other groups. If the stressors are internal, they see as the source inadequate socialization, failures in communication, or, by chance, as it were, insufficient resources—a condition that leads to scarcity's becoming a stressor. The stressors, in this view, are not really stressors, or rather they are stressors because we, the members of the group, see them as such. If we can learn to view things differently, to talk things through, to give up unrealistic demands, we will not have stressors.

My own commitment is to a conflict model of social processes (meaning not that I like it better but rather that I think it explains reality more adequately). Over and above the exogenic, accidental stressors, I suggest, are stressors that are inherent in the nature of all intragroup and intergroup processes. An individual family, a social movement, a social class are, by their very natures, confronted with both internal and external conflict. This is not to say that the stressors found in a family that is stable are of the same order of magnitude or of the same content as those found in a family with multiple problems. Black and white, poor and rich differ. But the difference is, as I have put it earlier, between a seriously moderate level of stressors and the level of almost constant emergency. It is, I contend, therefore absurd to search for the explanation of high group levels of health ease in the direction of the absence of stressors.

Character of Tension

In the early part of this chapter, I pointed to what seemed to be an emerging consensus about the transactional character of stressors. In 1974 I wrote, "But if anything has been learned in the study of stressful life events, it is that what is important for their consequences is the subjective perception of the meaning of the event rather than its objective character" (Antonovsky, 1974, p. 246). In this chapter, I have argued that this position is accurate but not important, in large measure because all of us confront what we define as stressors much of our lives. What, then, is the response of the organism to a confrontation with stressors? Overwhelmingly, the literature posits a state of stress. I suggest instead that it is of the utmost importance to distinguish between two states that I have proposed (Antonovsky, 1971) be called tension and stress.

Selye originally defined the stress syndrome as consisting of all the nonspecifically induced changes in response to stressors. He more precisely defined it as the well-known, three-stage general adaptation syndrome: alarm reaction, resistance, and exhaustion. Selye was careful to underscore that these were stages in adaptation. Evocation of the alarm and resistance stages, he suggested, and even of the stage of exhaustion, provided it is reversible, need not be damaging to the organism. "In the course of a normal human life, everybody goes through these first two stages many, many times. Otherwise we could never become adapted to perform all the activities and resist all the injuries which are man's lot" (Selye, 1956, p. 64). But, in his most recent clarification, he goes one step beyond suggesting the functional, positive consequences of the response to stressors. "With more recent sophisticated methods it is possible to show that essentially the same syndrome is also elicited by demands for adaptation, experienced as agreeable or beneficial; these are designated as 'eustress' in opposition to 'distress'" (Selye, 1975, p. 39).

Unfortunately, it is not quite clear what is "experienced as agreeable"; is it the demand—the stressor? Is it the emotion accompanying the stages of the adaptation syndrome or the consequences of the stress situation? Nor do I find that the literature is of much help. Stressors, by and large, are presumed to be bad: we are unhappy when we encounter them; the physiological and biochemical changes in response to stressors are accompanied by unpleasant affect; and the ultimate consequences are sad. Here and there one finds qualifications. Holmes and Masuda (1974) insist that the important thing about stressors is the adaptive demand made on the organism, irrespective of whether the life event is happy or sad. They disregard affect and are concerned solely with negative consequences. Most often those who are committed to the transactional approach point out that with adequate preparation, adequate coping skills, and resources, there is no stress: "Most life situations are not experienced as threatening because they do not tax people's capacities." But if we are not prepared to cope, then we will experience "anxiety, fear, depression, general discomfort" as a result of having been "exposed to some stress situation"—that is, "physical, social, and cultural conditions likely to be discomforting." (Quotes are from Mechanic, 1968, pp. 304, 299, and 297.)

Quite in contradistinction to the overwhelming emphasis in the field (though not to hints here and there) I suggest that: (1) The definition of stressor given in the early part of this chapter carries no implication of any necessary value judgment by the person or group confronting the stressor. (2) The response of the organism to a stressor—a response I propose calling *tension*—can be accompanied by either or both negative and positive affect. (3) The consequences to the organism of having entered a state of tension can be negative, neutral, or salutary.

In order to clarify this position, let us take as a possibly homey example moving one's family residence, particularly when the move is to a new community. Millions of Americans move each year. Anyone who has ever moved surely will agree that, by and large, it is quite a stressor. Weissman and Paykel (1972) conducted a most interesting study of the relationship between moving and depression in women. They note that moving often involves financial burdens and risks, loss of familiar people and habits and sights and involvement with new ones, technical problems including breakage and loss, and energy drain. The stressors are clear, and there is no doubt that we enter a state of tension—that is, the first two stages of Selye's general adaptation syndrome and possibly even the third stage, with all the biochemical, physiological, and emotional accompaniments. But what are these emotional accompaniments? They may well be, as was the case for the women studied, negative. But they need not be. One may feel excitement, exhilaration, challenge, relief—not because everything about the move was smooth sailing, not because one felt no tension, not because the demands were not defined by one as stressors. Moving unquestionably taxes people's capacities, in Mechanic's terms. "The stressful effects of American geographical mobility," Weissman and Paykel (p. 28) conclude, "have been underestimated. Moving often places inordinate demands on the individual to adapt and raises continued challenges to his identity. . . . There are a substantial number of persons who do experience incapacitating suffering." But this only after they have noted that "many people move each year and experience no problems or only transient ones."

The point, I trust, is clear. Tension is aroused by stressors. But we can be delighted or pained—or, for that matter, both simultaneously—by the tension. This point begins to be understandable if we consider the frequency of the voluntary search for stressors. I am not referring to masochistic tendencies, nor am I concerned with the acceptance of tension as a price to be paid in order to achieve a goal. Possibly the root is in what many posit as a fundamental exploratory urge. Others have spoken of the wish for new experience. The pattern may be related to the earlier-discussed unpleasantness of underload. Whatever the source, human beings constantly choose to enter stressful situations—in bed, in football matches, in risk-taking ventures—not only as a gamble for ultimate drive reduction but for the sheer pleasure of the tension. (See Radloff and Helmreich, 1968, for a detailed study of people who voluntarily enter a situation with a high stressor load, exploration of the continental shelf.)

The term *drive reduction* can take us to the next step. I have argued that tension per se can be pleasurable. But what are its consequences? It is not only inadequate but misleading to say, Well, if drive reduction is reasonably quick, if homeostasis is rapidly regained, or, as I prefer to put it, if tension management is efficient —no harm done. The consequences of a state of tension can be not only unharmful but indeed salutary. Perhaps the most forceful example that has come to my attention is found in what my colleague Shuval (1957–1958) calls the hardening hypothesis. In her study of the adjustment of concentration camp survivors to the rigors of Israeli life in the early 1950s, she found that survivors, under certain conditions, were better adjusted than those in control groups. Their point of reference for current difficulties was the horror they had somehow managed to overcome. The exercise model is another case in point. We place a special load on ourselves by demanding more than routine, automatic energy response, and we foster the emergence of possibly hitherto unknown capacities. We learn, and we can apply such learning to future stressors. The point need not be belabored because it is so familiar in everyone's experience.

I would like to borrow from another field the term that seems to me to apply perfectly to the possible salutary consequences of tension. In a report of some rat experiments, we read, "In summary, we have shown that environmental stressors not only can depress immune responsiveness but can also enhance it. Both suppression and potentiation [are possible]" (Monjan and Collector, 1977, p. 308). *Potentiation*—the calling up of hitherto potential resources and thereby enriching one's repertoire—is precisely a possible consequence of tension. One might go even a step further and posit protection as a positive result of tension. The consequences of initial exposure to microorganisms are too well known even to be cited. As another example, "the development and toleration of . . . anxiety is not only inevitable but also desirable both as a stimulus to early infantile development and as an essential prerequisite for the construction of adequate defenses in all danger situations" (E. R. Zetzel, quoted in Roazen, 1968, p. 281).

Tension, then, must be distinguished from stress. Stress is a contributing factor in pathogenesis. Tension can be salutogenic, but it also can lead to stress. Unless a distinction is made between the two concepts, this connection cannot be seen. When the distinction is made, the next crucial question can be asked: What determines whether a state of tension will be transformed into a state of stress or will have neutral or salutary consequences? Or, in the frame of reference of this book: What determines whether a person in a state of tension will be pushed in one direction or the other on the health ease/dis-ease continuum? The phrase I have used (Antonovsky, 1971, p. 1580) in dealing with this question is *tension management,* "defined as the rapidity and completeness with which problems are resolved and tension dissipated." Consideration of the possible salutary consequences of tension, however, suggests that the word *rapidity* may be misleading. Sometimes tension may be resolved so quickly that it prevents full beneficial consequences. Thus, for example, premature ejaculation can be most unsatisfying; compulsory arbitration to avoid a strike may prevent full clarification of the underlying issues. With this caveat, the crucial question becomes: What are the determinants of successful tension management? The answer I have suggested is found in the construct of resistance resources.

Let me conclude this chapter by quoting from Vickers' discussion of the mismatch between "symbolic representations of what is happening and of what 'ought' to be happening" (Vickers, 1968, p. 358): "A model of conflict does not necessarily tell us anything at all about pathological stress. Conflict is endemic; breakdown is still, happily, relatively exceptional. We need not—and therefore must not—assume that conflict in itself is noxious. . . . We need to understand both the noxious nature of a given stress in relation to the organization of a given organism and the vulnerability of a given organism to a particular form of stress. That, of course, involves an elaboration of the conceptual model far ahead of anything on which I have yet touched." We now turn to consideration of what I propose as a second major element in such a model.

Chapter Four

Tension Management
and Resources
for Resistance

If bugs are ubiquitous, endogenic in human existence, and extremely resourceful; if we are all subjected to a constant barrage of what we ourselves would define as stressors or to those bugs that, though not in the forefront of our consciousness (such as microorganisms, unconscious conflicts, and strivings or social pressures), we would quite readily agree to call stressors were we aware of them; if levels of tension and imbalance range from moderate but real to unimaginably high for different individuals and subcultures; if tension is not at all necessarily pathogenic; and if the data indicate that a surprising number of us indeed manifest pathology at any one time—then the crucial question becomes, How do we manage tension and prevent it from leading to stress? What are the resources at our disposal that enable some of us or, rather, all of us, as long as we are alive, to resolve tension at least some of the time?

Meaning of Resistance Resources

In my paper for the 1973 Stressful Life Events Conference (Antonovsky, 1974), I referred to resistance resources as "the most exciting things to be studied." I was far from being alone in taking this position. A pathogenic orientation, however, particularly within the framework of the traditional medical model of the single bullet, immunological or therapeutic, pressures one to focus on specific resistance resources relevant to a particular disease. Even when, under the influence of Selye's concept of the general adaptation syndrome, I formulated the breakdown concept of dis-ease, I was still tempted to think in terms of particular diseases. Not until I had developed a salutogenic orientation—at first about "deviants" such as those concentration camp survivors, poor people, or members of minorities who do stay at a fairly high level of health ease and then, in view of the ubiquity of stressors, about everybody—did I become aware of the full significance of generalized resistance resources (GRRs). Only then did I appreciate what I myself had written (Antonovsky, 1972, p. 541): "Because the demands which are made on people are so variegated and in good part so unpredictable, it seems imperative to focus on developing a fuller understanding of those generalized resistance resources that can be applied to meet all demands." At the most general, preliminary level, I defined a GRR as any characteristic of the person, the group, or the environment that can facilitate effective tension management.

This is not to deny the importance of specific resistance resources. They are many and are often useful in particular situations of tension. A certain drug, telephone lifelines of suicide-prevention agencies, or an understanding look in the eyes of an audience to whom one is lecturing can be of great help in coping with particular stressors. But these are all too often matters of chance or luck, as well as being helpful only in particular situations. One can go even further. It is the GRR that determines the extent to which specific resistance resources are available to us. Thus, if I may anticipate, being literate or being rich—which I see as a GRR—opens the way to exploitation of many specific resistance resources—for example, knowing one's way around a hospital bureaucracy.

One further preliminary point should be made. Rejection of the health/disease dichotomy opens the way for application of the GRR concept to all people at all times. Whatever one's location at a given point in time on the health ease/dis-ease continuum, the extent to which GRRs are available to one plays a decisive role in determining movement toward the healthy end of the continuum or, at least, holding one's own.

In my initial exploration of the GRR concept, writing largely intuitively, I identified three kinds of general resistance resources: adaptability on the physiological, biochemical, psychological, cultural, and social levels; profound ties to concrete, immediate others; and commitment of and institutionalized ties between the individual and the total community. The approach made sense to me. It seemed to fit some data, particularly epidemiological. The job of research, then, was to move from the intuitive to the systematic consideration of the GRR concept. The remainder of this chapter is devoted to this enterprise.

Avoidance of Stressors

As a point of departure, we would do well to consider that type of generalized resistance resource that is essentially "negative" in character: preventive knowledge, attitudes, and behavior. This resource is employed in order to avoid—or, more accurately, has the consequence of avoiding—exposure to stressors. The emphasis of Chapter Three on the ubiquity of stressors was not at all meant to suggest that individuals and groups do not differ in exposure to stressors. One of the reasons for such differences is the differential distribution of the GRRs that enable one to avoid exposure.

The most directly pertinent GRR of this type is what has been called a preventive health orientation. Briefly put, Rosenstock and his colleagues have hypothesized that persons with this orientation are likely to engage in behavior that, in our terms, helps them avoid stressors: they are vaccinated against polio; they have preventive dental and general medical checkups, breast examinations, Pap smears, and so on (Rosenstock, 1960; for a critical development of this approach, see Mechanic, 1968, pp. 130ff., and Antonovsky and Kats, 1970).

But this GRR is of interest in even more general terms. Essentially, it is the underlying concept of preventive medicine, of the health care orientation, of the philosophy so cogently expounded by McKeown (1976). In part, the approach is oriented to specific diseases, but this is not necessarily the case. Not smoking, eating a balanced diet, engaging in physical exercise are essentially to manage tension, in our terms, by not getting into a state of tension—that is, by avoiding stressors.

Let me be clear that I in no way denigrate this approach (much as I do not at all denigrate the traditional medical model). The society or community that adopts the Medizin-Polizei approach, in the more traditional public health terms in democratic societies or in the more extreme terms in totalitarian societies, will undoubtedly chalk up significant gains in the health of its population. The evidence of past and present is strong. On the individual level, there is also no doubt that prevention and early detection pay. But we are often prey to enthusiasm unwarranted by the data, as expressed in some material of the cancer societies (see Antonovsky and Hartman, 1974, for an evaluation of the efficacy of early detection). The cholesterol controversy points to a second problem, that of arriving at action proposals without adequate knowledge (Cochrane, 1972a). It often strikes me that converts are a danger to a good cause. They tend to become true believers, thinking that X is the total, instant solution to the only problem that matters. Not only does this single-mindedness alienate others from considering X; it sometimes inhibits any serious evaluation of the efficacy of X. A good current example is physical exercise and jogging in particular. I would predict that the religious enthusiasm now found will have to confront the double-edged consequences that this X might have.

A third problem of the preventive approach consists in ignoring the price paid for adopting a health care, risk-avoidance action as if health care were the only human value. Consider the financial cost of many screening tests or health education programs that utilize scarce resources without adequate evaluation and weighing of alternative resource allocations. Or consider the price in anxiety of people whose constant question becomes, "Is it bad for my health?" Or consider the more serious price of the medicalization of human existence, professional control, and government intervention. These caveats notwithstanding, there is no denying the importance of the preventive health orientation based on the concept of the avoidance of stressors.

Having said this, one must add that limitation of the GRR concept to this one area would be most unfortunate. Even in Samuel Butler's *Erewhon* the bugs were smarter. People became ill. Moreover, much of the advice often given to potential victims is gratuitous and insulting: "Don't moonlight. Take the family on a relaxing vacation. Don't eat so many starchy foods. Don't walk in darkened areas where you may be raped." Over and above the misplaced ideological implications of blaming the victim, the changes in life style are often forced on us by the social organization within which we live and in which individual choice plays only a minor role.

GRRs, then, undoubtedly have the one function of avoiding stressors. This discussion of avoidance of risk factors, as it is usually called, is brief only because it has already been considered so much more adequately than I could possibly do, particularly by McKeown (1976). What has not, in my view, been adequately discussed is what happens when, as is inevitable, stressors are not avoided and tension is created? What GRRs are available to manage tension?

Systematic Consideration of GRRs

Two factors have shaped the following discussion of GRRs. First, it has been guided, both in organization and in content, by a simple mapping-sentence definition of a GRR. The second factor is even more compelling, namely, my own limited knowledge of the extant literature I believe to be relevant. But, as will be seen at the close of the chapter, it is not particularly important that the mapping sentence is inadequate or that not every profile has been considered or that an important reference has been omitted. The crucial question, as will be seen, will become, What do these GRRs have in common? What is it that makes them GRRs? I do hope, however, that the mapping sentence in Table 6 is of some help at least for organizing the material.

Table 6.   Mapping-Sentence Definition of a Generalized
Resistance Resource

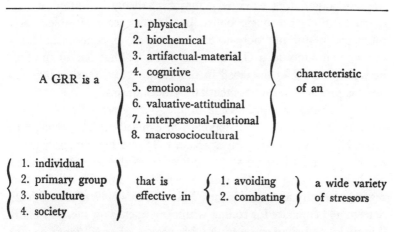

and thus preventing tension from being transformed into stress.

Physical and Biochemical GRRs. I have, perhaps unwisely, not refrained in earlier chapters from including physical and biochemical agents under the rubric of bugs, or stressors. Having thus been foolhardy, I believe no further harm can be done by at least briefly alluding to GRRs at this level.

The concept of immunological surveillance is closely associated with the work of Burnet (1971, pp. 131, 151ff.). His particular concern has been with cancer. Thus he writes of "a surveillance function perpetually patrolling the body, as it were, for evildoers." Elsewhere he speaks of the "complex mechanisms . . . [that] police the body for any abnormal mutant cells which by developing toward malignancy threaten survival." But he seems to go somewhat beyond this in discussing aging, where he implies an even more general resistance resource: "a fading-out of maintenance. . . . Nature loses interest after age x." Unfortunately, he does not discuss just what he means by "maintenance" or "nature." In a more recent paper with the same focus, we read (Oettgen, 1977, p. 488): "Agents such as BCG and *C. parvum* are known to increase immune responsiveness to a variety of antigens, and they can be counteracted by immunosuppressive measures. It seems likely that they affect the growth of antigenic tumors by raising the general level of immune responsiveness and so are aptly named immunopotentiators. . . . The determination of how immunopotentiators work is a major challenge." Indeed it is. I mean to imply no magic bullet, but it does seem possible that it might be useful not only to immunologists to conceptualize immunopotentiators as a GRR. It may well be that one of the links between the GRRs discussed in this chapter and tension management is precisely immunopotentiating mechanisms.

Dobzhansky quite some time ago suggested a genetic basis for human plasticity: "Genotypes are evolved which permit their possessors to adjust themselves successfully to a certain spectrum of environments by homeostatic modification of the phenotype." If indeed this proved to be the case, it would certainly be legitimate to regard plasticity as a significant GRR. The existence of a genetically determined capacity for rolling with the punches or, more formally, "plasticity of behavior under a wide variety of conditions" cannot, however, be proved "at this time by observation or experiment" (1955, p. 345; see also Lerner, 1968, p. 231).

Dubos has, possibly more than anyone else, focused on adaptability as humankind's most distinctive characteristic. "The plasticity of man's nervous system enables him to make a wide range of behavioral adjustments without having to depend on the slow process of biological evolution" (1973, p. 95). This neurological departure from tropismatically shaped, inflexible responses to stimuli is one of the distinguishing features of the human species. Some other species may have found far more comfortable ecological niches or, in present terms, environments that pose far fewer stressors than those confronting human beings. It may well be that our choice of environment, our "commitment," was unwise on the part of our species. Having made it, however, we are dependent on plasticity as a vital GRR. This is not to say that plasticity of the nervous system is a completely clear, objectively definable, and measurable characteristic. The significance of the concept, much as of other GRRs discussed here, is that it opens up avenues of research.

This neurological departure leads us directly into the area of more particular concern and prominence in this book: the psychological, social, and cultural GRRs available to people and groups in coping with stressors. If we are endowed innately with such plasticity, our lives would be most chaotic, Dubos points out, were our behavior (in the broadest sense) not ordered, constrained, and guided by culture and society. Much as the bugs that confront us are no less psychological and sociocultural than physical and biochemical, so the GRRs available to us are in all domains.

But before turning to a discussion of these GRRs, let me explain what may seem to be a remarkable omission. Selye, one of the leading figures in stress research, is the originator of the construct of the three-stage general adaptation syndrome: alarm reaction, resistance, and exhaustion. The term *generalized resistance resource* seems to suggest that the second stage is most germane to our discussion. Yet a close examination of Selye's description of this stage (1956, especially pp. 87ff.) reveals that one must make an important distinction. The GRR concept refers primarily to characteristics that facilitate dealing with and overcoming the stressor. Selye's concern, in his discussion of the resistance stage, is with actions of the organism that are directed at containing and offsetting the expressions of the alarm reaction, in order that the organism not enter the third stage of exhaustion. Thus resistance, in Selye's terms, does not relate to coping with the stressor. It is, as it were, a holding action, designed to prevent damage in the hope that the stressor will somehow go away. Selye's 1975 paper confirms the distinction made here.

The approach of Wolff and his colleagues, who have made such a major contribution to the stress field, is similarly largely not pertinent here (Wolf and Goodell, 1968). Again, their concern is with how the body reacts to a "circumstance of threatening significance to the organism," in the sense of the etiology of bodily diseases and disorders. This focus is likewise characteristic of psychosomatic medicine in the tradition of Alexander (1950). To reiterate: Our concern is not with the important question of how the body copes with the biochemical and physiological expressions of tension but with those GRRs that are applicable to the stressor directly and that function to resolve the problem set by the stressor.

Artifactual-Material GRRs. At the outset of our consideration of psychological, social, and cultural GRRs, I would pay explicit attention to one GRR. With all our sophistication, we often overlook the obvious. In extended discussions of coping with stressors, one seldom finds reference to wealth. A search not only in my own memory and work but in the indexes and texts of some of the major publications on stress reveals no reference to material resources as a GRR. The overwhelming emphasis in the literature is on the stressors confronted by poor people. Bound by the pathogenic orientation, we think in these terms.

Access to money, the symbolic equivalent of resources, is, I suggest, an important GRR in all societies. Money buys a safe abortion to deal with the stressor of an unwanted pregnancy. Its possession may assuage ego conflicts. Not only does money directly facilitate coping with stressors; but, linked to the acquisition of other GRRs, it also is indirectly powerful. In some societies wealth matters less than in other societies; in some historical and social situations the possession of money may be a stressor. Whether we like it or not, however, these are quite unusual exceptions.

Reference to money allows us to consider an issue that, though seemingly methodological, is a central theoretical issue applicable to many GRRs. Is there, we might ask, a simple linear correlation between a GRR and success in coping with stressors or is there a qualitative leap beyond a given level? In my work on social class and overall mortality (Antonovsky, 1967b), I suggested—again, pathogenically oriented—that the data indicated that the lower-lower class was significantly different from other classes. Is it the case that those who are wealthy enough, in J. P. Morgan's classic phrase, not to have to ask how much a yacht costs have a GRR that is qualitatively different from the money GRR of the rest of us?

It is superfluous to extend this discussion of material resources as a GRR. Two further points of clarification, however, are necessary. First, it is wise to distinguish analytically between material resources and interpersonal relations. Material resources are money, physical strength, shelter, clothing, adequate food, and the like. Interpersonal relations include power, status, availability of services. Second, in order to assess the significance of a given type of material GRR, one must know the particular culture. In one culture or subculture, physical strength may be a potent weapon in coping with stressors; in another, money may be more effective.

Cognitive and Emotional GRRs. It would be both unnecessary and impossible to canvass the entire psychological literature to identify important intrapersonal cognitive and emotional GRRs. I therefore limit the discussion here to two characteristics: knowledge-intelligence and ego identity. This limitation has the virtue of allowing the discussion to remain on the appropriate level of generality rather than entering the domain of specific traits and skills. Further, it covers both the cognitive and emotional domains, implicitly indicating the direction of further research in identifying intrapersonal GRRs. (I have intentionally excluded from the present discussion certain conceptualizations that focus on personality, in particular those of George Engel and his colleagues, of Eleanor Wertheim, and of Martin Seligman. I have excluded them here because of their crucial importance, on a higher order of abstraction, to the central thesis of this book. Thus discussion of these approaches is reserved for Chapter Five. This point is also applicable to the discussion below of sociocultural GRRs and the work of Melvin Kohn.)

Knowledge-intelligence as a GRR is used here in the broadest cognitive sense to encompass both a storehouse of information about the real world and skills that facilitate acquiring such knowledge. In modern societies, knowledge-intelligence is to a considerable extent contingent on literacy and formal education; in more traditional societies, the skill that is best called wisdom is the central component of knowledge. The specific reference here is to a fund of information—to stick to the above examples, about smoking-cancer data, techniques of contraception—and the skill that facilitates acquiring such information. One might equally well speak of knowing about Tay-Sachs disease and amniocentesis or, for that matter, about medicinal herbs. Or, to go one step further, of knowing about (and knowing one's way about) community services, opportunities, and rights. Of no less importance is the cognitive skill that enables one to distinguish between quacks or fakers and healers. Elsewhere, I have suggested that one of the reasons one finds a generally inverse relationship between social class and mortality is the differential availability of knowledge and cognitive skills (Antonovsky, 1968; Antonovsky and Bernstein, 1977). The examples given are from the health field, but many others might well be given from other areas. By and large, we find that those individuals and groups who possess knowledge in one realm are likely to possess knowledge in other realms of life (Caplovitz, 1963, especially chap. 12; Knupfer, 1947). This overlap of knowledge allows us to speak of knowledge-intelligence as a GRR.

I have no illusions that knowledge-intelligence is the decisive GRR in coping with stressors. The inordinate difficulties and, by and large, the failures of health education based on a cognitive approach are painfully familiar. Even though I know the epidemiological data well and am of reasonable intelligence, I still smoke. I have pointed out to many physicians enthusiastic about sex education the futility of teaching about reproductive physiology in the attempt to help adolescents cope with sexual stressors. Knowledge-intelligence, nonetheless, is seldom a handicap in coping; it often goes hand in hand with more potent weapons, and occasionally it may be decisive.

On the emotional level, the central concept is ego identity, which I regard as a crucial GRR. Again, the literature is vast, and I have selected a small part for discussion.

Like many other commentators with an essentially pathogenic orientation, Schachtel (1962) starts his discussion by focusing on the extreme of nonidentity: the number of the concentration camp inmate or the paper identity of the person in a bureaucratic social system. Schachtel goes on to speak of someone who lacks identity as having a sense of being an impostor, of wanting to hide something important about oneself, consciously or not, or of not having something one ought to have that would make one a real person. One travels, as he puts it well, with a false passport. One yearns for an identity that is real, inner, acceptable, and stable. Pain leads one to seek things to build up one's ego, to make one feel good. Schachtel wisely points out that this public image version of the ego is the "most important model of an alienated concept of identity." One grabs hold, as it were, of some fixed characteristic, role, or relationship, insisting that this is the fixed I. The result of adopting this reified concept of the ego is that one cuts oneself off from the dynamic, real world. This is true no less for those with a positive than for those with a negative, alienated identity concept. Assuming a fixed role, in the present context, makes it impossible to cope with stressors. Dorian Gray, in Schachtel's final image, is hopelessly lost; a picture is inevitably impotent.

I have opened the discussion of identity as a GRR with Schachtel's nonidentity because it so well offsets the essence of meaningful ego identity. To further explicate, we turn to Erik Erikson (1960, pp. 47, 49): "Identity *formation* neither begins nor ends with adolescence; it is a lifelong development largely unconscious to the individual and to his society, . . . an *evolving configuration*—a configuration that is gradually established by successive ego syntheses and resyntheses— . . . integrating *constitutional givens, idiosyncratic libidinal needs, favored capacities, significant identifications, effective defenses, successful sublimations, and consistent roles*" (emphasis in original). It would take us too far afield to follow Erikson in his profound discussion of the relationship between ego identity and social roles, group membership, and ideology, and its function as a basis for intimacy, generativity, and integrity. For our purposes, the central elements of ego identity as a GRR have been indicated: a sense of the inner person, integrated and stable, yet dynamic and flexible; related to social and cultural reality, yet with independence, so that neither narcissism nor being a template of external reality is needed.

Two further points are indicated. First, in much of the literature on mental health, a strong ego identity is taken to be the equivalent of mental health. This, it seems to me, is an expression of the confusion and difficulty in defining the term. Mental health is a more complex issue than is ego identity. But even if the two were accepted as identical rather than as dependent and independent variables, this identity would be of little help in explaining the location of a person on the health ease/dis-ease continuum.

The second issue is central to the thesis of this book. Chapter Five develops the concept of a sense of coherence. Clear distinction must be made between this concept and the concept of ego identity. Ego identity refers to a picture of oneself; the sense of coherence, to a picture of one's world, which, of course, includes the self. It may well be that a strong ego identity will turn out to be a decisive, or even a necessary, precondition for a strong sense of coherence. I trust that the distinction between the two concepts will become clear in Chapter Five. For the time being, I simply take note of my view that a strong ego identity is a GRR and not the equivalent of a strong sense of coherence.

Valuative-Attitudinal GRRs. Heretofore, we have focused on essentially intraindividual factors that characterize individuals and that they may bring to bear in coping with a variety of stressors. We now move to consider what have usually been called coping styles. These too are individual characteristics, but they are best understood when they are seen, to use Lazarus' term, in a transactional context.

A note of caution is in place. Our cultural preconditioning tends to prejudice us to assume that what may be called a mastery coping style or orientation is ever and always the only effective and respectworthy style of coping with stressors. One question raised about the Holocaust is, Why did Jews behave like lambs led to the slaughter? Only those who understand Jewish history are capable of appreciating that a central component of Jewish culture, developed over many centuries of harsh experience, was a mode of coping quite different from that of a mastery orientation. This other mode was extraordinarily effective for survival. That it may not have been appropriate in the face of the unique and utterly incomprehensible Nazi program of genocide—much as no other mode of coping could have been appropriate—is beside the point. In discussing cultural GRRs below, I shall return to this issue. For the present, it is appropriate simply to call the reader's attention to our cultural bias.

Unfortunately, there is little clarity in the concept of coping. Sometimes it is confused with the outcome of an interaction with a stressor. Thus, for example, Shalit (1977) studied the characteristics of tasks that facilitated or inhibited coping, in the sense of resolution of a problem. Rahe (1974, p. 74) takes a similar but narrower position in defining *coping* "as one's abilities to reduce his physiological activation, . . . such as a subject's ability to relax, and thereby alter his psychophysiologic activation"; he refers to the successful outcome of dealing with a physiologic problem, whatever its cause. However, many writers do view coping as a behavior pattern of dealing with a problem. Whatever one does, then, becomes a coping pattern. Thus Roeske (1978), in discussing how women deal with hysterectomy, writes of "normally controlled and usually assumes the leadership" (p. 15) as exemplifying one coping pattern and using "illness to attract attention and extract sympathy" (p. 18) as another such pattern. Anything, then, can be said to be coping—a view that hardly clarifies the concept.

Lazarus, one of the leading workers in the field of coping with stressors, has made major contributions to conceptual clarification. Let us, then, examine the Lazarus-Cohen transactional model of stress (1977), focusing on the second and particularly the third of its five key features: cognitive appraisal and coping. In Chapter Three, I noted that cognitive appraisal referred primarily to the meaning of the stressor for the person. But one aspect of cognitive appraisal is germane here: "the individual's judgment of the coping resources available or of vulnerabilities in the face of given dangers" (p. 111). In describing the coping processes, Lazarus and Cohen write: "Most persons . . . utilize a variety of coping strategies, anticipating and evaluating what might happen and what has to be done, planning and preparing, changing the environment, retreating when necessary, postponing action for maximum effect, tolerating frustration and pain, and even deceiving themselves in order to feel better and to maintain hope and a sense of self-worth" (p. 112). Let us overlook the lack of clarity in including "judgment . . . of vulnerabilities" in cognitive appraisal and "evaluating what might happen" in coping strategies. What is of greater concern and relevance is that Lazarus and Cohen, in their eagerness to reject seeing coping as a fixed "structural property of a person," throw the baby out with the bath water by implying that there is a necessary contradiction between a transactional model of stress and a systematic analysis of coping modes. Such systematic analysis would be much more helpful than an endless list of coping modes or actions.

We should, however, heed Lazarus and Cohen's warning that people use different coping strategies contingently, that is, in relation to the particular stress situation within which they are acting. If, however, the thesis of Chapter Three is accurate—that we all live at a moderate to high level of confrontation with stressors—then there is some basis for thinking that, given our individual cultural, historical, structural, and personal-historical backgrounds, we each tend to work out a typical coping strategy. This proposal is, I submit, consistent with the transactional approach.

The task before us, then, is to specify the appropriate patterns of alternative coping strategies that do not violate the recognition that coping strategies are always conducted in a historical-cultural as well as in a situational context. But the task is even more difficult. Our entire discussion is based on the premise that we can identify coping strategies that serve as GRRs. This identification requires ranking according to effectiveness. Unfortunately, as far as I know, we can obtain little help from the empirical literature. The attempt, then, must be viewed as a proposal subject to testing and not one based on evidence.

Let us define a coping strategy as an overall plan of action for overcoming stressors. One traditional way of categorizing coping strategies is the fight-flight-freeze triad. Scott and Howard (1970) reformulate this category with more sophistication, using the terms assertive, divergent, and inert responses. For descriptive purposes, this approach may be useful. But if we wish to identify the coping strategies that are effective GRRs, such classification is misleading. Despite our cultural prejudice in favor of fighting (at least for males), clearly an assertive response is not always the most effective strategy for coping with stressors.

I would point to three major variables that enter into every coping strategy: rationality, flexibility, and farsightedness. These, I suggest, are not situation-contingent characteristics. The more a coping strategy is high on these variables, the more effective a GRR it will be.

Rationality here is the accurate, objective assessment of the extent to which a stressor is indeed a threat to one, given who one is, in the broadest sense. To adopt a transactional approach—to stress the meaning of a stimulus to the perceiver—is not to deny objective reality. At one extreme, one's rational definition of a situation is decisive in determining the outcome. The objective observer would indeed say that a student who freezes in examinations is being rational in defining the examination as threatening (assuming it is important to the student to pass the examination). But in many situations a coping strategy is irrational, in that there is a totally inaccurate assessment of the stimulus and of who one is. The Jew in Germany in the 1930s who saw himself as immune; the teenage girl who considers the chances of becoming pregnant as a result of intercourse as nil; the person who pooh-poohs the data on smoking and lung cancer are not thereby guaranteed immunity. To put it simply: The importance of W. I. Thomas' dictum "If men define situations as real, they are real in their consequences" has not been fully understood. One's definition of the situation does not necessarily transform the reality, though it may. (Compare Petrie's 1967 discussion of a genetically determined tendency to be an "augmenter" or a "reducer.")

Flexibility refers to the availability of contingency plans and tactics and of a willingness to consider them. Given the dynamic character of coping with stressors, the strategy that is open to constant, built-in evaluation and subsequent revision—that is open to new information—is bound to be more successful, other things being equal, than other strategies. Note that receipt of new information and readiness to change one's course does not mean that one necessarily will do so. Nor does it mean that action is perpetually postponed, pending new information.

The third element of a coping strategy that contributes to making it a GRR is *farsightedness,* or, if one wills, being a good chess player. Farsightedness is linked to rationality and flexibility but goes beyond them in that it seeks to anticipate the response of the environment, inner and outer, to the actions envisaged by the strategy. The most rational and flexible coping strategy for our student may be to steal a copy of the examination and at the same time pay a fellow student to cooperate in cheating. But the coping strategy will be more effective if he anticipates the pangs of conscience or what will happen if he is caught, weighing these as additional data in deciding on behavior (see Mechanic, 1962).

To avoid misunderstanding, I should add that a coping strategy is a plan for behavior, not the behavior that eventually results to cope with the stressor. Such behavior is shaped by many variables, including coping strategies. Further, I would remind the reader that our concern is not with the substance of a strategy for coping with a given stressor at a given time. I have posited the possibility of an enduring, general coping strategy that is characterized by a high level of rationality, flexibility, and farsightedness. Such a coping strategy, I suggest, is an important GRR.

It may well be that emotional affect is a fourth important characteristic of a coping strategy. Lowenthal and Chiriboga (1973) suggest that some people prototypically respond to stressors by feeling overwhelmed, while others are challenged. I doubt that this is the case for more than a few people, though many might show a tendency in one direction or the other. More important for present purposes, however, I see no basis for arguing that such an overall tendency is consistently functional. Unlike rationality, flexibility, and farsightedness, one cannot say that the more one tends to perceive a stressor as a challenge, the more effective is one likely to be in coping with the stressor. It puts Don Quixote in mind.

Interpersonal-Relational GRRs. We now come to what may be the most substantiated and promising field of relevant research. It has more often than not been called social supports. For a long time, particularly in the area of mental health research, the pathogenic orientation led to a focus on social isolates, on those who might be called social destructs. Only recently has attention been paid at least to the entire continuum and, here and there, to what, in the present context, I would call the GRR of deep, immediate interpersonal roots.

Let me start by selectively calling attention to a number of studies that shed light on social supports. Gove (1973) has analyzed cause-specific mortality data and has shown the protective function that simply being married plays, particularly in relation to those causes of death where one's psychological state plays a direct or indirect role. He further reports, however, that being married is much more advantageous, in this sense, for men than for women. A paper by Phillips and Feldman (1973) analyzes the dates of death of famous people in relation to their dates of birth and of Jews in pre-World War I Budapest in relation to Yom Kippur. In each case a significant dip in deaths was found before the ceremonial occasion. The authors, in my view correctly, hypothesize that the occasion marked a reaffirmation of the social ties of the individual to a group. Hochschild (1975) takes this issue even further in her theoretical reanalysis of disengagement theory, suggesting that social and psychological disengagement is generally much more proximate to death than we generally think.

Probably the most recent and thorough analysis of the relationship between social supports and health outcomes is that of Berkman (1977). In 1965, data had been collected on a random sample of adults in Alameda County, California. The 682 persons who died in the following nine years, out of almost 7,000 persons in the sample, were identified. Included in the original data were four measures of social ties: marriage, close friends and relatives, church membership, and informal and formal group associations. Each of the four factors predicted mortality independently. A social-network index, combining all four measures, showed that people with many social contacts had the lowest mortality rates. This association was found to be controlling for a variety of sociodemographic and risk-factor measures. Though Berkman's concluding formulation focuses on "the hypothesis that isolation and lack of social and community ties may influence host resistance and increase vulnerability to disease in general" (p. 3), her findings are completely consistent with a salutogenic formulation; such ties can be viewed as GRRs. One might go further and postulate that if isolation and lack of ties are crucial, they can best be understood as a stressor. We would then anticipate a qualitative leap between the mortality rates of isolates and the rates of all others. Instead, we find a linear association, which suggests that social ties are indeed a GRR; it is not only their absence that matters. (See also Cobb, 1976, for a review of studies of social supports.)

Finally, mention should be made of the Israeli menopause studies (Datan, Antonovsky, and Maoz, forthcoming), reviewed in the Introduction to this book. It will be recalled that in designing the study of ethnic differences in the adaptation to climacterium, we had anticipated a linear relationship between the modernity-traditionalism continuum and successful adaptation. We differed on whether the most traditional women (Israeli Arab village women) or the most modern women (Israeli Jewish, middle-class urban women of central European origin) would be best or worst adapted, using a wide variety of measures of adaptation. Instead, we found (to summarize the findings in overall and necessarily oversimplified

terms)' a curvilinear relationship. The European women, closely
followed by the Arab women, were the best adapted; the North
African, Turkish, and Persian women adapted much more poorly
in the climacteric period. The most powerful explanation we could
present is germane in the present context. The content, styles, roles,
statuses, norms, and contexts of the lives of the European and of the
Arab women differed considerably. But what both groups of women
shared, by and large, was being embedded in networks of relatively
stable social relationships and in coherent, relatively integrated
subcultures.

The most adequate concept, I would suggest, that subsumes
the findings of much of the work that deals with interpersonal-relational GRRs is that of commitment. The pathogenic orientation has
led to a fairly extended consideration of the complex concept of
alienation. A salutogenic orientation leads us to focus on commitment. (The idea that commitment is the quite unexplored opposite
end of an alienation-commitment continuum is proposed in Antonovsky and Antonovsky, 1974.)

In a totally different context, Kanter (1968) has given us
what seems to me to be the most adequate theoretical analysis of
the concept of commitment. She defines commitment as "the
process through which individual interests become attached to the
carrying out of socially organized patterns of behavior which are
seen as . . . expressing the nature and needs of the person"
(p. 500). She identifies three analytically and empirically separable,
though interdependent, types of commitment. Continuance commitment is essentially a cognitive judgment that it is worthwhile for one
to remain within a group. Consciously or not, we balance the profits
and losses and arrive at a tentative conclusion. Cohesion commitment refers to a cathectic orientation, the extent to which one feels
affective ties to one's group and to its members. Identification, solidarity, and gratification from interpersonal interaction are part of
this dimension. Control commitment is an evaluation along the lines
of good-bad of the legitimacy of the group, the moral rightness of
the group's norms, its ways of doing things, its authority structure,
its goals, and its means for their achievement.

The extent to which one is embedded in social networks to
which one is committed, I suggest, is a crucial GRR. I am fully

aware that it is a complex, multidimensional concept, not at all easily made operational. Moreover, one must be aware of a crucial hidden assumption: If I am deeply committed to a given network and to its members, does this necessarily mean that the group or people in it are necessarily reciprocally oriented? In order that commitment serve as a GRR, such reciprocation is crucial.

I would add one further point here on an issue that has befuddled much of the literature on alienation. In our study of the kibbutz (Antonovsky and Antonovsky, 1974), we pointed out that one must distinguish between alienation-commitment with reference to primary and to secondary groups. There is no necessary contradiction between having extremely strong commitments to one's family, friends, work group, or other primary groups and extreme alienation from larger social structures such as community, union, social class, and nation. The two must be considered separately, which most of the measures of alienation certainly do not do. For present purposes, however, our concern is, as indicated by the subheading of this section, with those immediate social settings in which daily life is lived.

Macrosociocultural GRRs. This distinction can serve as a transition to our consideration of the last type of GRR. My temptation is to stop here and refer the reader to Malinowski's classic article on culture, which appeared in 1931. The article discusses the fundamental points I would make here more adequately than I could hope to do. Let me, then, summarize these points as they relate to salutogenesis and generalized resistance resources on the macrosociocultural level.

In essence, Malinowski says that culture gives each of us our place in the world. We are given (or learn to acquire) a language in which to communicate, a role set and a norm set, and a larger world in which to fit (or not fit). In Chapter Three, I defined a stressor as a demand made on one for which one does not have an automatic and readily available response capacity. From this point of view, what culture does, in giving us our place in the world, is to give us an extraordinarily wide range of answers to demands. The demands and the answers are routinized: from the psychological point of view, they are internalized; from the sociological point of view, they are institutionalized.

But what happens when, as is inevitably the case, life remains full of stressors? Or, to put it another way, what happens when cultures fail to provide routinized answers, as all cultures do, inherently and inevitably, to some extent or other? Does a culture make generalized resistance resources available to individuals and groups? This, then, is the present crucial question. As Malinowski answers it: "But however much knowledge and science help man in allowing him to obtain what he wants, they are unable completely to control chance, to eliminate accidents, to foresee the unexpected turn of natural events, or to make human handiwork reliable and adequate to meet all practical requirements. . . . In this field . . . there develops a special type of ritual activities which anthropology labels collectively as magic. . . . The richest domain of magic, however, is, in civilization as in savagery, that of health" (pp. 634–636).

Magic, however, "is distinguished from religion in that the latter creates values and attains ends directly, whereas magic consists of acts which . . . are effective only as a means to an end." But religion too is, in our terms, a GRR: "Religious belief and ritual, by making the critical acts and the social contracts of human life public, traditionally standardized, and subject to supernatural sanctions, strengthen the bonds of human cohesion. . . . Religion in its ethics sanctifies human life. . . . It grows out of every culture, because knowledge which gives foresight fails to overcome fate; because lifelong bonds of cooperation and mutual interest create sentiments, and sentiments rebel against death and dissolution" (p. 642).

One might go on in this vein, as Malinowski does, to discuss play, secular rituals, mythology, and artistic expressions of society as well as ideologies and philosophies that Malinowski, oriented to preliterate societies, tends to disregard. But there is no need. The point, I take it, is clear: At one ideal pole of the continuum, not to be remotely approximated in human history, a culture provides its members, group and individual, with ready answers, clear, stable, integrated; with keening for a death, an explanation for pain, a ceremony for crop failure, and a form for disposition and accession of leaders. At the other extreme, which at times becomes a reality for individuals and groups, there is only utter chaos; there are no answers. Ready answers provided by one's culture and its social structure are probably the most powerful GRR of all.

Absence of a GRR as a Stressor

Before we move on to integrate the concepts discussed in this chapter, it is important to point out a fundamental characteristic of GRRs. Throughout, I have considered them as resources; that is, I have viewed a GRR as something which, in the possession of a group or individual, makes possible either the avoidance of stressors or the resolution of tension generated by stressors that have not been avoided or both. I have seen a GRR, then, as something that one has, as something that characterizes one.

But there is another way of looking at the matter with respect to some GRRs. What happens when one is low on a given GRR? One possibility is that of substitutability. Merton (1968, pp. 86–91) has warned us of the danger of that variant of functionalism that assumes that if consequence X is a function of phenomenon A, then A must be maintained if one wishes X to be maintained. Thus, for example, if social cohesion is strengthened by religious homogeneity, religious homogeneity is viewed as essential to social cohesion. It would take us too far afield to explore the question of substitutability of GRRs, but we should keep it in mind. The implication of the question in the present context will, I trust, become clear in the pages that follow, in which the relation of GRRs to the sense of coherence is considered.

But even if we assume that a GRR can be substituted for another in managing tension, we must note that the absence of some GRRs can become a stressor. Perhaps the simplest example is that of money. Although having money obviously does not solve all problems, it helps with many. But not having money is not simply a matter of not having a given resource at one's disposal. Being in such a circumstance often directly and immediately is a stressor. Not only is access to need satisfaction blocked. But also the knowledge that one is penniless is a source of anguish in and of itself—a situation that can hardly be appreciated by those who have never been in such straits.

In Chapter Seven we shall consider the particular problem

of circularity in the central model of this book. It will there become clear that a given location on the breakdown continuum not only is a consequence of other variables but also serves as a GRR (if one is high on the scale) or as a stressor (if one is low).

Keeping these examples in mind, I would ask the reader to reconsider the absence of GRRs discussed in this chapter as possible stressors. In keeping with my salutogenic orientation, I have not raised this issue until the present. It would, however, have been misleading to have totally neglected its consideration.

GRRs as Providers of Negative Entropy

Consideration of the absence of a GRR as a stressor opens the way for further development of the phenomenon under review in this chapter. In Chapter Three, I suggested that the ubiquity of stressors in human existence is analogous to the Second Law of Thermodynamics; it points to an inevitable increase of positive entropy, or disorder. But unlike the closed systems with which the law deals, the human organism is an open system. The input of negative entropy may well be adequate, at any given point in time, or even over a longer period of time, to offset the inherent tendency to disorder. It strikes me that it may be extremely useful to view the period of early childhood as one in which the input of negative entropy from the external environment or, in Schrödinger's (1968) vivid image, particularly apt here, the "sucking of orderliness from [the] environment" is (or, rather, can be) sufficient to lower the level of positive entropy, of disorder, in the child. Is this not the essence of growth—the increasing orderliness of language, of muscle control, of interpersonal relations, and so on?

In these terms, is it not appropriate to see stressors, originating in either the internal or external environment, as entropic, increasing the level of disorder of the system? And to see GRRs, again whether originating in the internal or external environment, as negatively entropic, decreasing the level of disorder of the system?

If GRRs can be defined as characteristics that introduce negative entropy into the system, the mapping sentence (Table 6) needs to be modified. It is indeed quite useful in providing a systematic basis for considering a wide range of phenomena as possible

GRRs. It prevents the psychologist from thinking of ego identity and ignoring all else; it reminds the sociologist and anthropologist that they tend to forget genetics and immunology, and the biological scientists that the social scientists have a contribution to make. But, in the last analysis, inclusion of a generalized resistance resource for discussion in this chapter was intuitive, or if data suggested a correlation between it and tension management, inclusion was empirical. The mapping sentence is not yet a guide for determining whether a given phenomenon or characteristic is a GRR.

To put the matter another way, the mapping sentence does not provide a culling rule. It is essentially tautological, in that it states the criterion for inclusion as a GRR to be an empirical correlation with tension management. This criterion makes it impossible to test a hypothesis that a GRR facilitates tension management. It does not tell us why a phenomenon is effective in combating a wide variety of stressors.

We can resolve this problem by modifying the mapping sentence within the framework of the concept of negative entropy. Thus, a *generalized resistance resource* is a physical, biochemical, and so forth (see Table 6) characteristic, phenomenon, or relationship of an individual, primary group, subculture, society that provides extended and continued experience in making sense of the countless stimuli with which one is constantly bombarded and facilitates the perception that the stimuli one transmits are being received by the intended recipients without distortion. Making sense, in information theory, refers to the provision of information rather than noise. But, following Thomas, I would also include music. As Thomas (1974, pp. 22–25) writes: "It is one of our problems that as we become crowded together, the sounds we make to each other . . . become more random-sounding, accidental, or incidental, and we have trouble selecting meaningful signals out of the noise. . . . We are only saved by music from being overwhelmed by nonsense. . . . The need to make music, and to listen to it, is universally expressed by human beings."

This definition of a GRR, moreover, goes beyond providing a criterion for identifying GRRs. By providing a unifying theme, an overarching concept, it makes possible a resolution of the incredible complexity of stress research. In a review of this field from an interactionist perspective, Chan (1977) cites a wide variety of intrapersonal, interpersonal, and situational variables that, in our terms, would seem to be related to tension management. No degree of methodological and statistical sophistication, I suggest, will resolve the problem of which Chan (p. 100) writes: "disentangling the many intriguing complexities arising from the person-situation interaction." Only a more adequate theoretical formulation can do so.

Significance of GRRs

We can now, I propose, take the decisive step in formulating the significance of GRRs. The extent to which our lives provide us with GRRs is a major determinant of the extent to which we come to have a generalized, pervasive orientation that I call a strong sense of coherence.

In a paper that speculates about the possible exploitation of information theory in analyzing biological situations, Rapoport (1968) discusses Maxwell's Demon, whom he familiarly calls Maxie. Maxie is "a being whose faculties are so sharpened that he can follow every molecule in his course." He "works with 100 percent efficiency pumping information [negative entropy] into a system." A person with a sense of coherence, I suggest, is like Maxie, though it is inconceivable that any human being or social group can ever remotely approximate the theoretical efficiency of this improbable imp. The extent to which this approximation is realized, however, determines the efficiency with which tension is managed.

Chapter Five

Perceiving the World
as Coherent

The time has now come for a formal definition of the concept that integrates all the foregoing details, implicit and explicit, and that is a crucial variable in explaining movement on the health ease/disease continuum. The *sense of coherence* is a global orientation that expresses the extent to which one has a pervasive, enduring though dynamic feeling of confidence that one's internal and external environments are predictable and that there is a high probability that things will work out as well as can reasonably be expected. Almost invariably when I have presented this concept, people have had an immediate, intuitive response of "I know very well what you're talking about." In the particular cultural context in which the concept has been presented, it is often taken to mean "I am in control" and associated with the concept of an internal locus of control. This cultural bias is discussed in detail below. Once this misinterpretation is clarified, I have found that the concept makes important sense to people.

One of the reasons it does is that people can identify in their personal experience—both in their own lives and in their reading of literature—individuals with a strong sense of coherence as well as individuals with a markedly weak sense of coherence. Thomas Mann's vivid portrayal of Mynheer Peeperkorn in *The Magic Mountain* illustrates a strong sense of coherence. In *The Brothers Karamazov*, Fëdor Dostoevsky has given us a masterly contrast of the two extremes: Ivan and Dmitri Karamazov, each of whose sense of coherence is, in its own way, minimal compared with that of Alyosha. Perhaps the supreme example in literature, particularly appropriate because one individual moves from one extreme to the other, is that of Job.

Intuitive approval of a concept that is intended as an explanatory and hypothesis-generating tool, however, is only a starting point. It is crucial to analyze all the facets of the definition and to clarify possible misunderstanding and the precise implications of each of the terms.

Analysis of the Definition

As defined, the sense of coherence explicitly and unequivocally is a generalized, long-lasting way of seeing the world and one's life in it. It is perceptual, with both cognitive and affective components. Its referent is not this or that area of life, this or that problem or situation, this or that time, or, in our terms, this or that stressor. It is, I suggest, a crucial element in the basic personality structure of an individual and in the ambiance of a subculture, culture, or historical period.

This does not mean that there are no ups and downs. A particular experience, a specific situation, a detailed success or failure can effect a temporary and minor shift in one's sense of coherence. (In fact, being impervious to particular changes in one's environment is one indication of what I subsequently call a fake sense of coherence.) But such changes occur around a stable location on the continuum.

The term *dynamic* in the definition takes us much beyond such minor fluctuations. Its meaning will become fully clear, I hope, in the discussion below of the sources of the sense of coherence. I certainly am not committed to understanding the sense of coherence as being determined forever and anon by genes or early childhood experience. It is shaped and tested, reinforced and modified not only in childhood but throughout one's life.

To take an example. The pathogenic orientation, particularly in the hands of clinicians, clarifies the dynamic pattern of a deteriorating sense of coherence. Thus the psychotherapist seeks to point out to the neurotic patient how he or she continually gets involved in endeavors that by definition are doomed to failure; the psychotherapist then focuses on the sources of this neurotic pattern. He or she may even note how such continued experiences weaken the sense of coherence. A salutogenic orientation, however, can lead to working with the patient to engage in goal-oriented behavior that promises success, thereby strengthening the sense of coherence.

Similarly, a radical change in one's structural situation—in marital status, occupation, place of residence—can lead to a significant modification in one's sense of coherence. But in addition one's sense of coherence, strong or weak, plays a significant role in determining one's choice of remaining in or changing one's structural situation. Thus, to stick to the above example, the neurotic, with a weak sense of coherence, may choose to avoid the "danger" of entering psychotherapy. In this sense, one tends to choose situations that reinforce the level of one's sense of coherence.

The same dynamic approach can be applied to different areas of life. If experience in one area tends to weaken while experience in another area tends to strengthen one's sense of coherence, the person with a stronger sense will seek to change the area that weakens it, while the person with a weaker sense will gravitate toward that area. In this way, there is a constant albeit dynamic tendency toward consistency and generalization, stability and continuity.

Stability and continuity bring us to the crux of the matter. A strong sense of coherence involves a perception of one's environments, inner and outer, as predictable and comprehensible. In the image that has been and will be used often, it means that the stimuli that impinge on one are meaningful, as information or as music. Even more important than the immediate response, however, is the overall expectation that stimuli will continue to be meaningful. This is what one's world is seen to be like. Receiving stimuli is only one side of one's transactional relationship with one's world, however. No less important is the confidence that the stimuli one sends will be received without undue distortion. Thus, one's world has form and structure, is choate and comprehensible. We should take note of one frequent situation. We receive stimuli that are perceived as noise. The person with a strong sense of coherence locates the trouble outside himself; the stimuli are nonsensical. But in the case of the stranger or the migrant, people all around speak a language that makes no sense, but one knows very well that the impediment is in oneself.

If one understands what is going on, however, and if the world is seen as predictable, outcomes may still not fulfill needs. And a person with a weaker sense of coherence will indeed tend to anticipate that things are likely to go wrong. When things make no sense and are not predictable, it is difficult to expect that needs will be fulfilled, except by sheer luck or blind chance. One can clutch at straws; one can engage in privatized (not culturally routinized and ritualized) magic. But one remains without much hope. The person with a stronger sense of coherence is quite able to see reality, to judge the likelihood of desirable outcomes in view of the countervailing forces operative in all of life. One is not blinded by confidence. It is in this context that the phrase *as well as can reasonably be expected* has been included in the definition of the concept. Malinowski's (1931) Trobriander fishermen, even after having engaged in all the proper rituals prior to fishing in the open sea, know full well that the rituals are no guarantee against drowning or a poor catch.

To put the matter another way: A strong sense of coherence is not at all equivalent to feeling that everything in life is handed to one on a silver platter or that one has the Midas touch. Quite the contrary may even be true. Life may well be seen as full of complexities, conflicts, and complications—which one understands. Goal achievement may be seen as contingent on immense investment of effort. Moreover, one may be fully aware that life involves failure and frustration. The important thing is that one has a sense of confidence, of faith, that, by and large, things will work out well. Not that things will have a Hollywood happy ending. This is why the proviso "as can reasonably be expected" is added. A strong sense of coherence includes a solid capacity to judge reality.

What makes frustration, failure, and pain tolerable without vitiating a strong sense of coherence is, to introduce another crucial term, the perception of *lawfulness*. Job was shattered not because of his terrible suffering, not because almost all that he had was taken from him. When fate is capricious, when events are arbitrary, when there is no lawfulness—and not at all when there is no omnipotence—the sense of coherence is shattered. In this lies the terrible brilliance of modern totalitarianism, foreshadowed in Franz Kafka's *Castle*. One never knows when the doorbell will ring or for what reason.

The ideas of predictability and lawfulness may suggest too great an emphasis on the cognitive aspect of the sense of coherence. A belief in lawfulness does not necessitate intellectual understanding of the logic of the laws. An orthodox Jew even regards such an attempt as apostasy—a view that led to the excommunication of Spinoza. The intellectual task, as well as the emotional aspiration, is to know God's laws; the behavioral task is to obey them. The rank-and-file party member need not understand the laws of history; this is the realm of the leadership. It is enough to maintain one's faith in God or in the party in order to maintain a strong sense of coherence. Such faith makes everything comprehensible, at least affectively. It is when faith collapses that the sense of coherence dissipates. The Holocaust, violating all previously known lawfulness, thus posed a most torturing problem for believing Jews. An approximation of their problem is found in Crossman (1950), in which six well-known ex-Communists analyze their break with the party.

We can now take the final step in clarifying the definition of sense of coherence. It is of the utmost importance that I did not choose the more familiar phrase *sense of control*, which clearly implies and is overwhelmingly used as meaning "I am in control." This conceptualization reflects a superfluous cultural bias, an issue discussed below. A sense of coherence, as I trust has become clear, does not at all imply that one is in control. It does involve one as a participant in the processes shaping one's destiny as well as one's daily experience. The orthodox Jew, striving with all his might to obey the 613 commandments, is not at all passive. The Calvinist on whom signs of grace have been bestowed in response to his utmost effort has been extremely active. But this does not mean that it is they who are decisive in the outcome.

The crucial issue is not whether power to determine such outcomes lies in our own hands or elsewhere. What is important is that the location of power is where it is legitimately supposed to be. This may be within oneself; it may be in the hands of the head of the family, patriarchs, leaders, formal authorities, the party, history, or a deity. The element of legitimacy assures one that issues will, in the long run, be resolved by such authority in one's own interests. Thus a strong sense of coherence is not at all endangered by not being in control oneself.

Case Histories

In order to convey more adequately what is meant by the sense of coherence, I have chosen three case histories. The fact that two of them relate directly to health is not accidental. But since this issue is explored in detail in Chapters Six and Seven, it is not the primary concern here. We start with Norman Cousins (1976).[1]

In August, 1964, I flew home from a trip abroad with a slight fever. . . . I was hospitalized . . . [and had] tests, some of which seemed to me to be more an assertion of the clinical capability of the hospital. . . . I turned them [lab technicians] away and had a sign posted on my door saying that I would give just one [blood] specimen every three days.

I had a fast-growing conviction that a hospital was no place for a person who was seriously ill [because of bad] . . . sanitation, . . . sometimes promiscuous use of x-ray equipment, the seemingly indiscriminate administration of tranquilizers and powerful pain

[1] Reprinted, with Norman Cousins' kind consent, by permission from *The New England Journal of Medicine,* Vol. 295, pp. 1458–1463, 1976.

killers, more for the convenience of hospital staff, . . . the reg-
ularity with which hospital routine takes precedence over the rest
requirements of the patient. . . . Perhaps the hospital's most
serious failure was in the area of nutrition.

My doctor . . . was able to put himself in the position of
the patient. . . . We had been close friends for more than twenty
years. . . . We had often discussed articles in the medical press.
. . . He felt comfortable about being candid with me. . . . Dr.
Hitzig called in experts. . . . He leveled with me, admitting that
one of the specialists had told him I had one chance in 500.

All this gave me a great deal to think about. Up to that
time, I had been more or less disposed to let the doctors worry
about my condition. But now I felt a compulsion to get into the
act. . . . I had better be something more than a passive char-
acter. . . . I thought as hard as I could about the sequence of
events immediately preceding the illness. . . . I wondered whether
the exposure to the hydrocarbons, . . . individual allergy, . . . a
condition of adrenal exhaustion [when] . . . I was less able to
tolerate a toxic experience [could be the cause]. . . . Our last
evening in Moscow had been . . . an exercise in almost total
frustration.

Assuming this hypothesis was true [exposure to diesel and
jet pollutants at a time of adrenal exhaustion], I had . . . to re-
store what Walter Cannon, in his famous book The Wisdom of the
Body, *called homeostasis. . . . I remembered having read . . .*
Hans Selye's classic book, The Stress of Life. *. . . If negative emo-*
tions produce negative chemical changes in the body, wouldn't the
positive emotions produce positive chemical changes? . . . Even
a reasonable degree of control over my emotions might have a
salutary physiologic effect. . . . A plan began to form in my mind
for systematic pursuit of the salutary emotions. . . .Two precondi-
tions for the experiment: . . . medication [could not be] toxic to
any degree . . . [and] I would have to find a place somewhat
more conducive to a positive outlook on life.

With Dr. Hitzig's support, we took allergy tests and discov-
ered that I was hypersensitive to virtually all the medication I was
receiving. . . . It was unreasonable to expect positive chemical
changes to take place so long as my body was being saturated with,

and toxified by, pain-killing medications. I had one of my research assistants at the Saturday Review *look up the pertinent references in the medical journals. . . . The history of medicine is replete with instances involving drugs and modes of treatment that were in use for many years before it was recognized that they did more harm than good. . . . Living in the second half of the twentieth century, I realized, confers no automatic protection against unwise or even dangerous drugs and methods.*

Pain is part of the body's magic. . . . I could stand pain so long as I knew that progress was being made in meeting the basic need . . . [of] the body's capacity to halt the continuing breakdown of connective tissue. . . . I recalled having read in the medical journals about the usefulness of ascorbic acid. . . . Couldn't it also combat inflammation?

I wanted to discuss some of these ruminations with Dr. Hitzig. He listened carefully. . . . He said that what was most important was that I continue to believe in everything I had said. He shared my sense of excitement . . . and liked the idea of a partnership.

Even before we had completed arrangements for moving out of the hospital, we began the part of the program calling for the full exercise of the affirmative emotions as a factor in enhancing the body chemistry. . . . A good place to begin, I thought, was with amusing movies. . . . The nurse was instructed in its [the movie projector's] use. . . . So we took sedimentation-rate readings just before as well as several hours after the laughter episodes.

The arrangements were now complete for me to move my act to a hotel room. . . . The sense of serenity was delicious. . . . I found him [Dr. Hitzig] completely open minded on the subject [of ascorbic acid]. . . . It seemed to me that, on balance, the risk was worth taking, . . . to know whether we were on the right track.

There was no doubt in my mind that I was going to make it back all the way. Two weeks later, my wife took me to Puerto Rico for some sustained sunshine. . . . I must not make it appear that all my infirmities disappeared overnight. . . . But I was back at my job at Saturday Review *full time again. . . . Is the recovery a total one? Year by year the mobility has improved. . . . [I hit a] tennis ball or golf ball, . . . ride a horse, . . . play the Toccata*

*and Fugue in D Minor. . . . My neck has a full turning radius
again.*

*What conclusions: . . . The will to live is not a theoretical
abstraction, but a physiologic reality. . . . I was incredibly fortunate to have as my doctor a man who knew that his biggest job was
to encourage to the fullest the patient's will to live and to mobilize
all the natural resources of body and mind to combat disease. Dr.
Hitzig was willing to set aside the large and often hazardous armamentarium . . . when he became convinced that his patient might
have something better to offer. . . . The principal contribution
made by my doctor to the taming, and possibly the conquest, of my
illness was that he encouraged me to believe I was a respected part-
ner with him in the total undertaking.*

Even a quick reading reveals five striking characteristics of
the case. First, Cousins was quite ready to be a sharp critic of the
hospital: the efficiency of its organization; its level of adequacy in
sanitation, nutrition, and use of equipment; its concern for the
patient. Second, a remarkable patient-doctor relationship is revealed. They were long-time friends. The doctor served as liaison to
specialists, was honest, supported the patient's active orientation,
and "shared my sense of excitement . . . and liked the idea of a
partnership." Third, and perhaps most central, we note the definition of Cousins' own role, with an unusual set of norms for a patient: get into the act, assume responsibility for therapeutic decision
making, take initiative, participate in assembling data and reviewing literature, formulate hypotheses. "*We* took sedimentation-rate
readings." Fourth, we see that Cousins' nonpatient roles are relevant. He was familiar with medical literature. He had a staff to do
research for him. He could afford to be "hospitalized" in a hotel.
And, finally, we read of his attitude toward pain and the idea that
"the risk was worth taking."

His experience, I submit, is a marvelous example not so
much, as Cousins puts it, of a will to live, but of a total behavior
pattern shaped by an extremely strong sense of coherence, rooted
in a concrete social structure and cultural setting. More important,
this general orientation quite evidently characterized Cousins before
his unfortunate trip to the Soviet Union. Note that I do not claim

that his sense of coherence caused the happy outcome, just as it did not prevent the onset of his illness.

Let us look next at the case of Sigmund Freud. Max Schur (1972), Freud's personal physician from 1928 until Freud's death in 1939, wrote: "One of the aims of this study is to trace the gradual development of different responses used by Freud to prevent situations of great stress and danger from becoming traumatic and to discover the ways Freud utilized to achieve mastery without resorting to denial" (p. 40). Schur's work is indeed of the utmost relevance for us, particularly his discussion of the most critical and difficult—and least healthy—years (1892–1899) of the first half of Freud's life (chaps. 2 and 3). On the one hand, relative poverty and major responsibilities, a near total break at about age thirty-six with the professional world around him and his own past, a publicly known plunge into the most chaotic (and, to Vienna, most repellent) of worlds; on the other hand, his wife Martha's love and the friendship of Fliess, and an extremely strong sense of coherence.

Unlike the article by Cousins, Schur's work contains no brief selection that is appropriate here. I have, therefore, chosen an alternative, which comes close to the mark. In his Introduction to the abridged edition of Jones' *Freud* (1961), Lionel Trilling writes:[2]

There is yet a third reason for the interest that Freud's life has for us— . . . the style and form of the life itself, . . . the consonance that we perceive between Freud's life and his work. The work is large and ordered and courageous and magnanimous in intention; and of the life we can say nothing less.

Overtly and without apology, Freud hoped to be a genius. . . . The commitment to achievement of both his family and his culture was reinforced by the ethical style which a traditional education proposed. . . . A heroic English Puritanism joined with the ancient ideal of public virtue to confirm the necessarily more private but no less rigorous notion of how a life must be lived: with sternness, fortitude, and honor.

[2] Excerpted from the Introduction, by Lionel Trilling, to *The Life and Work of Sigmund Freud,* by Ernest Jones, edited and abridged by Lionel Trilling and Steven Marcus, © 1961 by Basic Books, Inc., Publishers, New York. Abridged from *The Life and Work of Sigmund Freud,* 3 volumes, © 1953, 1955, 1957 by Ernest Jones. My appreciation is extended to Diana Trilling and to Basic Books for their consent.

Freud's intellectual achievement must be thought of as a moral achievement. I have two things in mind saying this. One has reference to the courage of a man in middle life, with family responsibilities and a thoroughly conventional notion of how these must be met, who risked his career for the sake of a theory that was anathema to the leaders of his profession. . . .

The other thing I would imply by speaking of the moral nature of Freud's achievement is suggested by Freud's own sense of his intellectual endowment. With this he was never satisfied. . . . "I am not really a man of science, not an observer, not an experimenter, and not a thinker. I am nothing but by temperament a conquistador—*an adventurer . . . with the curiosity, the boldness, and the tenacity." . . .*

Freud's last years were his darkest. Despite the high demand he made upon life, despite his notable powers of enjoyment, he had long regarded the human condition with a wry irony; and now by a series of events the cruel and irrational nature of human existence was borne in upon him with a new and terrible force: the defections of two of his most valued collaborators . . . [and] the shadow of death—[friend and patron], . . . his beautiful daughter Sophie, . . . Sophie's son Heinz [for whom Freud had a special love]. . . . In 1923 he learned that he had cancer of the jaw. [He had] thirty-three operations. . . . For sixteen years he was to live in pain. . . . The prosthesis he wore was awkward and painful, distorting his face and speech. . . . He had, of course, no religious faith to help him confront the gratuitousness of his suffering. Nor did he have any tincture of "philosophy." He is as stubborn as Job in refusing to take comfort from words—even more stubborn, for he will not permit himself the gratification of accusing. *The fact is as it is. Human life is a grim, irrational, humiliating business—nothing softens this judgment. . . . Yet nothing breaks him and nothing really diminishes him. He often says that he is diminished, but he is not. He frequently speaks of his indifference, but the work goes on.* Civilization and Its Discontents *. . . appears when he is seventy-three. At his death at eighty-three he is writing his* Outline of Psychoanalysis. *He sees patients up to a month before he dies. . . .*

This heroic egoism is surely . . . the secret of his moral being. "Mit welchem Recht?"—*"By what right?" he cries, his eyes blazing, when he is told in his last days that when the diagnosis of cancer was first made, there had been some thought among his friends of concealing the truth from him. . . . Through all his years of very great pain—near the end he spoke of his world as being "a little island of pain floating in a sea of indifference"—he took no analgesic drug and only at the last did he consent to take aspirin. He said he preferred to think in torment to not being able to think clearly. Only when he felt sure that he had outlived himself did he ask for the sedative by the help of which he passed from sleep into death.*

All comment would be superfluous.

The sense of coherence, as I have suggested, is a concept that is applicable to groups as well as to individuals. One of the most striking illustrations is found in Brinton's (1965) analysis of similarities that characterized the prerevolutionary periods in England, the United States, France, and Russia. Brinton's portrayal of the ruling class on the eve of revolution (pp. 53–59) in contrast with the ruling class that rules and believes in its rule catches the essence of a weak and of a strong sense of coherence, respectively.[3]

What may be called the ruling class seems in all four of our societies to be divided and inept. . . . [Earlier, it was they] who seemed to lead dramatic lives, about whom the more exciting scandals arose, who set the fashion, who had wealth, position, or at least reputation, who, in short, ruled. . . . It seems likely that the great masses of poor and middling folk . . . really accept the leadership of those at the top . . . and dream rather of joining them than of dislodging them.

[Just before the revolutions] the ruling classes in our societies seem . . . to have been unsuccessful in fulfilling their functions. . . . A mixture of the military virtues, of respect for established ways of thinking and behaving, and of willingness to compromise, and, if necessary, to innovate is probably an adequate rough approximation of the qualities of a successful ruling class.

When numerous and influential members of such a class begin to believe that they hold power unjustly or that all men are

---

[3] Reprinted with permission from the book *The Anatomy of Revolution* by Crane Brinton, © 1965 by Prentice-Hall, Inc. Published by Prentice-Hall, Inc., Englewood Cliffs, N.J. 07632.

brothers, equal in the eyes of eternal justice, or that the beliefs they were brought up on are silly or that "after us the deluge," they are not likely to resist successfully any serious attacks. . . . [Their] decadence is not necessarily a "moral" decadence. . . . The virtuous Lafayette was a much clearer sign of the unfitness of the French aristocracy to rule than were Pompadour or even DuBarry.

The Russians here provide us with a locus classicus*. . . . Russian aristocrats for decades before 1917 had been in the habit of bemoaning the futility of life, the backwardness of Russia, the Slavic sorrows of their conditions. . . . [They had] an uneasy feeling that their privileges would not last. Many of them, like Tolstoy, went over to the other side. Others turned liberal and began that process of granting concessions here and withdrawing them there. . . .*

When those of the ruling classes who had positions of political power did use force, they used it sporadically and inefficiently. . . . [They were] more than half ashamed to use force and therefore used it badly.

Perhaps nowhere better than in France is to be seen one of the concomitants of the kind of disintegration of the ruling class we have been discussing. This is the deliberate espousal by members of the ruling class of the cause of discontented or repressed classes— upperdogs voluntarily sitting with underdogs. . . . It is necessary to point out that the existence of rebellious radicals in the upper classes is only one symptom. . . . [They] must be relatively numerous as well as conspicuous in a society in disequilibrium. They, and the wasters and the cynics, must set the tone for the class— . . . the same mixture of weariness, doubt, humanitarian hopes, and irresponsibility.

Except perhaps in America, we find the ruling classes in the old regimes markedly divided, markedly unsuited to fulfill the functions of a ruling class. Some have joined the intellectuals and deserted the established order; . . . others have turned rebels, less because of hope for the future than because of boredom with the present; others have gone soft or indifferent or cynical. Many, possibly even most, . . . retained the simple faith in themselves and their position which is apparently necessary to a ruling class. But the tone of life in the upper classes was not set by such as these. The sober virtues, the whole complex series of value judgments which

*guards a privileged class from itself and others, all these were out of
fashion.*

From Brinton's analysis of the disintegration of the ruling
classes in prerevolutionary periods, we can reasonably draw four
major inferences that can be applied in our context. First, though
the point is most clearly seen in considering a ruling class, a strong
sense of coherence can characterize any social unit, from the Jones
family to a neighborhood, a city, a region, or a country; from a
local voluntary association to an apocalyptic religious movement;
from underdogs to overdogs. Second, it is not the number of individuals in the group with a strong sense of coherence that matters
but, as Brinton puts it, who sets the tone. Concomitantly, in a group
with a strong sense of coherence, defection of individual members is
viewed as random, accidental, and a sign of the weakness of the
defectors. When defection is viewed as inevitable, continuous, and
with sadness, it is a sign of a disintegrating sense of coherence.
Third, whatever the particular culture of the group with a strong
sense of coherence, there is a firm commitment to a set of goals
(hazy as that commitment might be) and a set of means to achieve
these goals—means that are held to be not only legitimate but the
embodiment of morality. Finally, the future is perceived as inevitable: stable continuity into infinity for the overdog; unavoidable
subservience for the underdog.

Sources of the Sense of Coherence

In Chapter Four, I proposed that "the extent to which our
lives provide us with GRRs is a major determinant of the extent to
which we come to have a generalized, pervasive orientation that I
call a strong sense of coherence." The GRRs discussed in that chapter were considered in essentially an intuitive albeit ordered manner.
Not until the end of the chapter was the inductive question asked,
What is it that all these GRRs have in common? Only then could
the linkage be proposed between GRRs and the sense of coherence.
At this point, having defined and clarified the concept of
the sense of coherence, we can take a further and crucial step. The

discussion of GRRs in Chapter Four in good part ignored the question of the sources of GRRs. One acquired these resources—material, personal, cognitive, social, and so forth—to a greater or lesser extent, it could have been inferred, almost by happenstance. This, of course, is not the case. It is not at all accidental that certain individuals and social groups are likely to have a much stronger sense of coherence than others. Particular social-structural and cultural-historical situations are quite likely to provide the developmental and reinforcing experiences that result in a strong sense of coherence.

In this light we turn to a consideration of the work of Engel and his colleagues, Seligman, Wertheim, Kohn, Rose Coser, and Kardiner. Their work, encountered at various stages in the development of my own model, is important in clarifying the concepts of generalized resistance resources and the sense of coherence. By considering similarities, parallelisms, and differences among the various approaches, we can go to the heart of that most important question: What conditions are central in providing adequate GRRs to develop, reinforce, and maintain a strong sense of coherence?

Psychological Sources. The work of George Engel and his colleagues at the University of Rochester has been of great importance in advancing the unfortunately named field of psychosomatic medicine. Guided by a pathogenic orientation, they have developed the central concept of the giving-up syndrome, whose meaning is best summarized in their own words (Sweeney, Tinling, and Schmale, 1970, p. 378).

> The affective response of "giving-up," when it follows real, threatened, or symbolic loss of a highly valued form of gratification, tends to precede the onset or exacerbation of somatic as well as psychic disease . . . [in that it] allows or facilitates whatever disease potential or predisposition exists in the individual or environment to become manifest. . . . [It] includes a loss of self-esteem, a disruption in object relationships, a decrease in motivation, and an expectation that such a state may be enduring. . . . The "giving-up" reaction can be divided into two phenomenologically distinct subtypes, which are

best described by the terms *helplessness* and *hopelessness*. The qualitative differences between these affects are postulated to have developmental bases. Helplessness is defined as a feeling of being left out or abandoned where loss of gratification is perceived as caused by external events or objects. . . . With hopelessness . . . the individual feels that he alone is responsible for the loss and that there is nothing he or anyone else can do to overcome it.

Subsequently, Schmale (1972) reviewed the extensive research that had been conducted in clarifying the giving-up syndrome and its origins. In the same year, Engel and Schmale reformulated the basic concept in a profound endeavor to link it to the process of biological adaptation of organisms. They proposed the concept of conservation-withdrawal, "a basic biological anlage serving survival" that comes to be "reflected in the behavior and psychological experience of man." Giving-up is viewed as the "inner experience of the person in whom the conservation-withdrawal mechanism has been activated" (1972, p. 72). In brief, the argument is as follows. All organisms are confronted, periodically or by chance, with unfavorable environmental conditions, in which a withdrawal rather than an active response is highly adaptive and serves "an elemental survival function" (p. 64). Appraisal of the situation indicates "either a too intense input which cannot be assimilated" (overload) or "a deficient input which indicates unavailability of supplies" (underload) (pp. 68–69). In such cases, activity is not only fruitless but is a waste of scarce resources. We have, then, become biologically equipped with both response modes, activity and withdrawal. The hibernation mode, however is risky: The supplies taken in previously for repair, renewal, and growth are, after all, limited.

In essence, one who has adopted habitual withdrawal as a dominant mode of behavior is unable to take sustenance from the environment while existent supplies are rapidly exhausted. The affinity with the concept of the sense of coherence is quite clear (except that the focus is pathogenic). In our terms, withdrawal as a general orientation is a marked inability to be accessible to the information and music that one's environment might well be sending, or, putting it otherwise, an inability to utilize the GRRs that do exist as potentials or to develop GRRs.

The conservation-withdrawal response mode becomes a classic, habitual, dominant syndrome through the repeated experience, particularly in the first six years of life, of failure to master feelings of helplessness and hopelessness, to learn to give up when appropriate, and to internalize a characterological balance between activity and withdrawal (Schmale, 1972). The resulting lifelong orientation toward conservation-withdrawal is, in our terms, a weak sense of coherence. (The relationship of this approach to the work of Bowlby, 1977, on attachment theory is quite clear.)

There is considerable compatibility between the work of Engel and his colleagues and that of Seligman (1975). Seligman, however, is an experimental psychologist and developed his model in the framework of psychological learning theory. "Helplessness," he writes, "is the psychological state that frequently results when events are uncontrollable" (p. 9). He points to two crucial elements that determine helplessness. First, the individual responds to stimuli in a locked manner rather than in a voluntary manner (contingently), a response that can be affected by reward and punishment. Second, and more crucially, the outcome of behavior is seen as noncontingent on one's behavior. Learned helplessness "produces a cognitive set in which people believe that success and failure is independent of their own skilled actions" (p. 38). On the motivational level, it "undermines response initiation quite generally" (p. 36). One observes "the striking giving-up sequence." Emotionally, learned helplessness involves first a fear-protest stage and then a helpless-depressed feeling.

Seligman explicitly stresses that what is crucial is not failure per se but "the loss of control over reinforcements"; no matter what one does, the outcome—which may even be positive—is not perceived as contingent. The similarity found in Seligman's work to the sense of coherence becomes even clearer in his discussion of safety signals and relevant feedback (p. 121). Predictability is made possible by safety signals, even if the signal connotes an undesirable outcome. At least in our terms, there is information, not noise.

Seligman contends that learned helplessness has its origins in early childhood and in the continued experience of response-outcome independence. Referring to René Spitz' studies of maternal deprivation, he argues that what is crucial is not the deprivation of stimulation per se but the deprivation of synchrony between action and feedback. This does not, he points out, mean that such deprivation has an inevitable result. On the contrary, he notes that the experience of the child in coping with anxiety and frustration, if the child masters these stimuli by his actions, is essential in building immunity against learned helplessness. Children who for whatever reasons constantly experience an absence of controllability learn to expect that nothing they do matters.

Two crucial points in Seligman's work should be stressed. First, though he is never quite explicit, he seems to regard it as essential, if learned helplessness is to be avoided, that the environment be comprehensible, ordered, and consistent, whatever the content of the signals. If one never knows what is coming, one never knows how to organize one's behavior. Seligman does not quite commit himself to this view, however. On the one hand, his key notion is that of contingency; on the other hand, he stresses that experience in mastery is vital: "Objective control, however, is a necessary condition for the development of the perception of control" (p. 138). The matter of control brings us to the second point. Seligman's total commitment is to a body of work rooted in the internal locus-of-control concept, a totally unnecessary and confusing bias to which I return later.

I would make reference here to the work of Wertheim (1975, 1978), whose detailed analysis and reconceptualization of early child development make a considerable contribution to understanding the development of what she calls autonomy and competence. As she defines them, there is good reason to posit an affinity between them and the sense of coherence.[4] Her starting point is the assumption that, from the time of intrauterine experience, a "doing-undergoing" dichotomy always characterizes the "person-

[4] In a personal communication, Wertheim writes: "The concepts of autonomy and competence represent an attempt in this direction, akin to your 'sense of coherence.' My ultimate aim is to arrive at a conceptual understanding of 'anthropogenesis,' or the capacity to be 'human.' . . . In this context it may be necessary to ask whether 'anthropogenesis' is a necessary but not a sufficient condition of 'salutogenesis,' or both are merely different aspects of the same process."

significant other" system and the "person–physical environment" (including one's own body) system. "An adaptively optimal person-environment system should be characterized throughout life by an appropriate dynamic balance between the 'power' of the person and the 'power' of the environment" (p. 2). In the case of both autonomy and competence, which are parallel, interdependent, and dynamic processes, Wertheim writes of "age-, sex-, and culture-adequate control"—that is, judgment as to the adequacy of the autonomy and competence balances can be made only in a given context. Such judgment, however, "can be viewed objectively or subjectively. . . . In the former case, autonomy and competence are evaluated from the point of view of specific sociocultural and/or clinical criteria. In the latter, perceptual processes, which are treated as the critical intervening variable mediating the individual's subjective sense of autonomy and competence, are examined" (p. 2).

I have referred to Wertheim's work here not because she has an answer to the question "of the roots, optimal developmental conditions, and subsequent developmental course of autonomy and competence" (p. 6) but because she has, more than others, I think, emphasized a number of important points in seeking an answer. First, she insists on an interactional framework for understanding development; living is a matter of constantly working out and reworking out a modus vivendi with the relevant persons and environments. Second, she stresses that such persons and environments form systems, and she does not focus on action-reaction patterns between individuals. Third, she opens the way for avoidance of the cultural bind of identifying coherence with "I am in control" both by speaking of a "doing-undergoing" balance and by her insistence on "age-, sex-, and culture-adequate control."

Although Wertheim does refer to a lifelong process of reworking autonomy and control, her detailed analysis focuses on early (and often very early) child-environment system transactions. Thus we come away from her work, and from the work of Engel and Seligman, with the important understanding that childrearing patterns that place a premium on autonomy and competence, an appropriately balanced withdrawal-conservation response mode, and the opposites of the giving-up syndrome and of helplessness are highly relevant sources of a strong sense of coherence. But none of them probe the social conditions that foster or impede such childrearing patterns. Nor do they consider the conditions of adult life that reinforce or weaken the developmental directions set in early life, beyond making passing reference that this can happen. Childrearing patterns, one might think, are located in a sociocultural vacuum.

Social-Structural Sources. For sociocultural connections, we can turn to the work of Melvin Kohn. His professional career has included three seemingly different major areas of study: social class and schizophrenia, parental values and childrearing patterns, and the structural conditions of occupational life. Though Kohn himself has explicitly made the link among these three areas, not all who know his work are aware of the close relationship. The question of the source of the sense of coherence highlights the integral connection among them.

Let us start from Kohn's work on schizophrenia (1968, 1973, 1976a). He notes that almost all of the more than fifty studies on social class and schizophrenia have shown highest rates in the lowest social class. He proposes an explanatory etiological model that is based on the joint occurrence of genetic predisposition; a socially determined high level of stressors; and a particular socially conditioned, orientational cognitive-emotional system. This cognitive-emotional system is of particular concern to us here. The orientational system proposed by Kohn as being an etiological factor in schizophrenia is almost precisely the essence of a weak sense of coherence (1976a, pp. 179–180): "[The schizophrenic is characterized by] fearfulness and distrust and by a fatalistic belief that he is at the mercy of forces beyond his control and often beyond his understanding. . . . An orientational system predicated on conforming to the dictates of authority results in a perception of social reality that is too simplistic and fearful to allow the individual to take advantage of options that might present themselves. It is too inflexible to permit effective coping with precisely those problematic and stressful circumstances that most require subtlety, flexibility, and a perceptive understanding of larger social complexities."

Kohn, then, is describing a certain "perception of social

reality." His hypothesis, well supported by a considerable body of evidence, is "that the constricted conditions of life experienced by people of lower social class position" are most conducive to the internalization of the described orientational system. In the same way, he shows that the life conditions of persons in other social class positions are conducive to alternative orientational systems.

What are these conditions of life that are relatively more characteristic of lower-class persons? Here, I suggest, we must carefully distinguish between conditions of poverty and poverty in a given historical setting. Being poor in a stable, generally legitimized social structure is not as likely to produce the perception of social reality that Kohn describes as much as is poverty that occurs "when a stratified social and economic system is breaking down or is being replaced by another as in the case of the transition from feudalism to capitalism or during periods of rapid technological change . . . [or] imperial conquest . . . [or] detribalization" (Lewis, 1970, p. 69). Lewis puts his finger on the core of the matter when he says that "the lack of effective participation and integration of the poor in the major institutions of the larger society is one of the crucial characteristics of the culture of poverty" (p. 70). It is not that they are isolated from such institutions. But in all their contacts with such institutions they experience over and over again powerlessness, arbitrariness, and bewilderment, and, whichever way they turn, they are victimized, without any apparent rules. This is the experience of reality, and this is the image of reality that is built up. Moreover, such an image is hardly weakened by the truly extensive participation of the poor in such social institutions as the legal system, the military, or the public relief system. (For an interesting and relevant study using the Holmes-Rahe life change instrument, see Justice and Duncan, 1976. They describe the life of child-abusing parents as one of prolonged crises that constantly knock them over and in which "the unpredictability of all kinds of changes" is the key variable. They do not ask what orientation system evolves out of this kind of life experience.)

Without in any way diminishing the importance of understanding the conditions that deprive lower-class people of GRRs and shape a weak sense of coherence, I believe the pathogenic focus prevents us from a full understanding of the phenomenon.

It also blinds us from asking about those who, despite such conditions, do make it. We can move ahead by returning to Kohn's work. For the majority of people in the Western world, after all, daily life is not the unpredictable and nearly chaotic world of the very poor. As a matter of fact, Kohn's studies on the conformity/self-direction orientations, to which we now turn, by and large exclude the very poor. In his study on social class and parental values, Kohn writes (1969, p. 189): "The essence of higher social class position is the expectation that one's decisions and actions can be consequential. . . . Self-direction—acting on the basis of one's own judgment, attending to internal dynamics as well as to external consequences, being open minded, being trustful of others, holding personally responsible moral standards—this is possible only if the actual conditions of life allow some freedom of action, some reason to feel in control of fate. . . . Self-direction, in short, requires opportunities and experiences that are much more available to people who are more favorably situated in the hierarchical order of society."

Turning to the empirical examination of such opportunities and experiences led Kohn to the study of people's jobs. Within the established, institutionalized, and internalized daily routine, our major role activity takes up the bulk of our time and energy and shapes, more than anything else, our place in society, be we teachers, executives, houseworkers, machinists, or sanitation workers. How, Kohn has asked, does this routine shape our orientation?

Kohn's central variable is the substantive complexity of work: "the degree to which the work, in its very substance, requires thought and independent judgment" (p. 1). (This summary of Kohn's work and the quotations are based largely on an unpublished paper—Kohn, forthcoming. For the published work on these issues, see Kohn, 1976b, 1969; and Kohn and Schooler, 1978.) Kohn's concern is with "the impact of work on [a] sense of self and orientation to the rest of the world" (p. 3). It is crucial to understand that Kohn is concerned with the objective conditions of work and their effects on personality and not with one's awareness of such conditions. "Substantively complex work, by its very nature, requires making many decisions that must take into account ill-defined or apparently conflicting contingencies. . . .

[Complexity] is at the heart of the experience of work. More than any other occupational condition, it gives meaning to this experience" (pp. 8–9).

In some of the most sophisticated empirical work of which I am aware, Kohn has shown (for men and, more recently, for employed women) that the substantive complexity of one's work "has a strong, independent relationship to many facets of psychological functioning, a relationship stronger than that of any other dimension of occupation (subjective or objective) we have studied" (p. 10). Further, a follow-up study has shown that the "substantive complexity of work . . . has a causal impact on psychological functioning" (p. 10). Kohn does not deny that personality influences what occupation one goes into and how one molds one's job. His contribution is in showing that at the least "cognitive processes do not become impervious to environmental influence after adolescence or early adulthood . . . [or] well into mid career" (p. 15).

Although Kohn's investigation of causality has been limited to substantive complexity and intellectual flexibility, he feels that he has at least a strong prima facie case that the substantive complexity of one's work also is causally related to "values, self-conception, and social orientation" (p. 17) and particularly to the powerlessness, normlessness, and self-estrangement components of alienation. These are even closer to our concerns. As Kohn puts it (pp. 18–20): "Thus, men who do complex work come to exercise their intellectual prowess not only on the job but also in their nonoccupational lives. They become more open to new experience. They come to value self-direction more highly. . . . [Complex work strengthens] one's sense that the problems one encounters in the world are solvable and manageable . . . [increases] one's valuation of self-direction and one's tolerance of deviant belief." In an article closely related to Kohn's concerns, Coser (1975) analyzes the psychological-orientational implications of embeddedness in "complex role sets and differentiated roles." (Kohn, it should be noted, has put the emphasis on the conditions of work, stressing substantive complexity and seeing complexity of work with people as but one type of substantive complexity. Coser sees complexity of work with people, conceptualized in terms of role sets, as central and other types of substantive complexity as secondary. For present purposes in seeking the sources of the sense of coherence, both approaches should be taken into account.) Though Coser's central focus is on the self-estrangement component of alienation or, on the positive side, individuality, she also deals with the socially structured preconditions for "innovation, flexibility, reflection, and self-direction . . . and empathy." As she puts it (p. 259): "It is in a differentiated social structure, where individuals are segmentally involved, where they are encouraged to take distance and to articulate their roles and their thoughts, that people are able to develop that degree of individuation that goes together with rationality and flexibility. . . . Complex role sets and differentiated roles are not alienating restrictions on individuality; they are its basic structural precondition."

I have concentrated on Kohn's and Coser's work here because they, more than anyone else I know of, have been concerned with the socially structured conditions—embedded in a system of social organization defined more than anything else by the social class dimension (though this is by far not the only dimension)— that foster the orientation with which we are concerned. Working at a certain kind of job (Kohn) or occupying a certain kind of role-set complex (Coser) leads one to see the world as complex—as offering alternatives and choices, making sense in different ways, allowing considered rationality, facilitating planning, having room for one's own action. Certain people, they say, more than others, because of where they are socially located, continually have such experiences; over time, they come to see the world in this complex way.

Finally, brief mention must be made again of Kohn's work (1969) on parental values and childrearing patterns. Parents set frameworks of expectations within which their children grow up. Compared with almost all other areas of life, childrearing provides parents with the opportunity to exercise an enormous amount of power. They set the rules and have the wherewithal, to a considerable extent, to enforce these rules. Kohn is particularly concerned with the dimension of self-direction/conformity, which can be seen in a broad sense to be congruent with Kohn's conceptualization of the general orientation of the lower social class as described in his work on schizophrenia. Kohn is thoroughly aware of social class structure. He knows that in all societies one's social class is one of the key variables that determine one's daily existence. His concern with social class brought him to ask, What is it about social class membership that molds the way one looks at the world? and to focus on one important element that he calls the substantive complexity of the job. Kohn's overarching thesis, then, can now be stated. Engaged in a job that offers extensive substantive complexity (buttressed by Coser's complex role set), one comes to have an orientation that is one of complexity and flexibility, alternatives and self-direction, meaning, consistency, choice, and a sense that problems are manageable and solvable. This orientation comes to expression, above all else, in how one raises one's children. Childrearing in turn develops the orientation of the next generation—an orientation that guides them in shaping their own lives and in selecting alternatives (such as jobs of substantive complexity).

I have taken the liberty of extrapolating from Kohn's concept of the self-direction/conformity orientation to the concept of sense of coherence. In doing so, I may have gone too far, for there is a fundamental difference, though not a contradiction, between the two. Self-direction is consonant with a strong sense of coherence in a particular sociocultural context. The availability of options and choice facilitates rationality in coping. The existence of alternatives affords the luxury of failure; one can try a different tack. But such self-direction is contingent on living in a society that approves of a variety of ways of doing things. Further, if the world is to be seen as comprehensible, self-direction must be accompanied by a considerable degree of tolerance of ambiguity. In other societies, where self-direction is hardly praiseworthy, substantive complexity and tolerance of ambiguity may well be inimical to a strong sense of coherence. Kohn's essential contribution to the exploration of the sources of a strong sense of coherence, then, is twofold. On a general theoretical level, he has shown how social structure shapes orientation. In the particular Western societies he has studied, he has carefully delineated one particular pathway.

Before turning to a consideration of alternative cultural pathways, we should note a fundamental though not intrinsic shortcoming in Kohn and Coser's work—a shortcoming most germane to our present concern. In their discussions of complexity, they fail to note two conditions that are essential in allowing a high degree of complexity to contribute to a general orientation in which the world is seen as predictable and comprehensible. First, the complexity must not be overwhelming; the number of choices must be somewhat limited, the number of impinging factors comprehensible. Second, and related to the first, the resources available to one must be such as to make it possible, at least a considerable part of the time, to solve the problems confronting one with a reasonable degree of success.

In reviewing studies of sex differences in coping, Shalit (1977) found articulation (the ease with which concepts can be ranked and differentiated from each other) to be most potent in successful coping. Thus he suggests that providing presurgical patients with too much information hinders coping, whereas selective attention, which makes articulation simpler, strengthens cognitive control and helps coping.

The second precondition that is necessary if job complexity is to facilitate development of a strong sense of coherence—the availability of resources for problem solution—is considered clearly in a Swedish study of sawmill workers. Kohn found a high correlation between job complexity and control by the worker over the work process. The authors of the Swedish study, however, describe a situation in which this is not the case. As Frankenhaueser and Gardell (1976, p. 44) describe the objective characteristics of the job, it involves a "demand on the worker to make skilled and economically important decisions"—a characteristic that at least seems to be related to Kohn's job complexity. The sawmill workers, however, have to make these decisions "at a pace set completely by the machine system." Thus these workers were confronted both by too much job complexity (quantitative overload) and "too low a degree of personal control over the work process" (qualitative underload). In such a double bind situation, one's work experience cannot become a GRR, as the data from the study suggest.[5]

[5] The reader may have noted that, with the exception of a passing reference to employed women, the focus of this section has been on men. I

Cultural-Historical Sources. Consideration of Kohn and Coser has taken us beyond the psychological focus on childrearing patterns and led us to consider location in a social structure as no less important in shaping one's GRRs (and, by implication, the patterned, prototypical GRRs of social groups and categories of persons). Kohn's work has also provided a link between the adult and child, the sociological and the psychological. We can now go further by introducing a cross-cultural and historical dimension. The present thesis is that certain cultural and historical situations foster a strong sense of coherence.

The work of Kardiner (1939, 1945) in the development of the basic personality structure concept, though written over three decades ago, is still extremely valuable. "The basic personality type for any society is that personality configuration which is shared by the bulk of the society's members as a result of the early experiences which they have in common. It does not correspond to the total personality of the individual but rather to the projective systems, . . . the value-attitude systems which are basic to the individual's personality configuration" (1945, p. viii). Working largely in small preliterate societies, Kardiner and his colleagues developed a theoretical model that is useful in clarifying the issue of the sources of a sense of coherence. Briefly, and with oversimplification, let me present Kardiner's model by arbitrarily taking as a starting point a given natural environment. People enter this environment and work out a culture and social structure, a set of answers to the fundamental problems of social existence. Among these answers is a prototypical family structure and childrearing patterns. Given the high order of coherence on the institutional and behavioral level throughout the society, the child is socialized in a particular direction that is most appropriate to, that fits best into, that society's social organization and culture. There is a hierarchy of systems in the basic personality structure, ranging from profound, unconscious

---

would point out that the theory of job complexity and control over job process can be applied directly to the major role activity of anyone: worker, housewife, pensioner, prisoner, patient, student. Unfortunately, the literature on male workers predominates. I know of only one serious study of the situation of the housewife that lends itself to this analysis (Oakley, 1975). Goffman's (1961) study of total institutions is certainly also germane, though again the focus is pathogenic.

projective systems through learned systems to pure empirical reality systems. Cutting across all these are value systems and ideologies (p. 34).

Having constructed this ideal-typical theoretical model, Kardiner then applied it to a number of concrete societies. His concerns were essentially two, and these are of direct significance to us. First, he asked, what is the content of a given basic personality structure in a given society? As a collaborator with anthropologists, he was able to systematically dispose of the notion that there is a fixed human nature. Each culture develops its own relatively stable human nature. For our purposes, this formulation raises the crucial question of whether different human natures—in the sense of different basic personality structures—are more or less consistent with a strong sense of coherence. I would go further and suggest that the sense of coherence is a major component of the basic personality structure.

Kardiner's detailed analyses of the Comanche and Tanala cultures (p. 99) point to two remarkably different culture patterns. In Comanche culture, group solidarity is based on the ego strength of the individual, the absence of segmental vested interests, the prohibition of overt expression of tension, and full cooperation without subordination. Among the Tanala, group solidarity is built about obedience and passivity, with fixed statuses, vested interests, and protection of the weak by the strong. These cultures are radically different from each other, but in both cases a consistent, lifelong experience that one's culture has clarity and consistency and makes sense leads to what I infer is a strong sense of coherence. These cultures are in extremely sharp contrast to the culture that occupies the bulk of Kardiner's book, the Alorese, whose essence can be summed up briefly (pp. 228ff.): "the low range of affectivity, the distrust, the low aspiration level, the amorphous aggression patterns, the limited capacity for strong attachments, the sensitivity with all varieties of defenses it mobilizes, the repressed predatory trends, . . . complete absence of anything that can be called government or even status, . . . complete lack of systematization." Clearly, this culture is not likely to place at the disposal of its members a considerable store of GRRs.

Kardiner's second central concern may be even more germane to us. All human beings live in a changing world. When, because of a change in climate and topographic conditions, the dry method of rice production became obsolete, all of Tanala culture underwent a radical change. "In Tanala we see a society which under one set of conditions had strong stability and through the change of subsistence economy became extremely unstable by virtue of the enormous amount of mutual hostility unleashed by the new economy" (p. 418). What is crucial for us here is not the earlier-noted issue (that some cultures are "better" than others for a strong sense of coherence) but that radical change and instability are, by their nature, not conducive to a strong sense of coherence.

In the last section of his study and in a subsequent study of American Negroes (Kardiner and Ovesey, 1951), Kardiner sought to apply his concepts to complex societies. In historical perspective, dealing with the emergence of capitalist industrial societies, Kardiner considers the basic personality structure "required by" such societies and best exemplified by Calvinism. Though it is tempting, it would take us too far afield to explore the Calvinist basic personality structure and its relation to a strong sense of coherence. Fromm (1941) has done this far more adequately than would be possible here. His concept of social character is no less an appropriate conceptual tool in analyzing cultural-historical sources of the sense of coherence than is Kardiner's basic personality structure. In this context, too, useful reference can be made to Erikson (1958), where we read (p. 263): "The answer lies in man's capacity to create order, which will give his children a disciplined as well as a tolerant conscience and a world within which to act affirmatively."

The importance of Kardiner's work (as well as that of Fromm and Erikson) for the present study is that he gives us the historical and cross-cultural perspective needed in order to gain an understanding of the sense of coherence. He leads us to ask two fundamental questions: To what extent does the society or subculture under consideration require a basic personality structure that involves a strong sense of coherence? And, no less important, to what extent does it provide a clear cultural image of the world, whatever the content of the image may be?

I do not see how it is possible to exaggerate the importance of the last point. Predictability and comprehensibility are the central themes of all the approaches we have considered. They are necessary albeit not sufficient prerequisites for the development of GRRs. Beyond this, we can specify additional conditions. What I trust has become clear in this lengthy exposition is that specifiable social conditions—certain specifiable childrearing patterns and subcultural and cultural patterns of social organization—provide a continued series of experiences that build up the GRRs that are crucial to a strong sense of coherence: a strong constitution, money, a clear ego identity, a flexible coping style, social supports, and so on. Over and over again, these GRRs allow us to see our internal and external environments as meaningful, predictable, and ordered. With this perception, we can reasonably hope that we can emerge victorious much of the time, though not necessarily in every encounter. It allows us to develop an orientation at whose core is "I (or we) can overcome."

I would be the last to claim that our knowledge is sufficient to specify the precise conditions under which a strong sense of coherence emerges. There is a great need for detailed research, both on the individual and on the group level. I should like to think, however, that the framework provided here allows us to formulate research questions—the key to any meaningful research. Let me give but one example. It strikes me that one common substantive theme that is shared by all the studies we have considered, from Engel's giving-up complex to Kardiner's Calvinist man, is the continuous experience of participation in shaping one's fate. How, we might ask, is such participation related to GRRs and to the sense of coherence?

Danger of Bias

This last point brings us to a most important issue that has been touched on here and there but has not been fully explored. Since Rotter published his monograph (1966), a significant amount of research has been conducted on his locus-of-control concept. Much of the work has been summarized in Lefcourt's book (1976) and most recently in an important paper by Perlmuter and Monty

(1977). Because of its similarity to the concept of the sense of coherence and because many of the readers of this book are familiar with this body of work, I find it most important to point up the fundamental distinction between the two concepts. (See the exchange of letters between myself and Perlmuter and Monty in Antonovsky, 1978.)

Rotter's fundamental distinction is between an internal and an external locus of control. Someone with an external locus of control has "the pervasive expectancy . . . that rewards and punishments do not occur because of one's own actions but are due instead to forces outside of one's control such as fate, luck, chance, or powerful others" (Naditch, 1974, p. 111). An internal locus of control, by contrast, locates one's fate in one's own hands. The tendency is most ethnocentrically powerful to equate sense of coherence, sense of control, and internal locus of control, using the model of the autonomous individual extolled in the litany of Western societies since the Industrial Revolution—or, perhaps more appropriately, the Protestant Reformation. This ideological paradigm dominates our own lives and shapes our science.

My point can be seen by reference to the first example given by Seligman (1975, chap. 1) to illustrate his definition of controllability. He first describes the behaviors of a competent, almost certainly suburban American housewife who smoothly and appropriately handles the quasi-emergency of her five-year-old's suffering a gash in the leg. That night the child's fever rises and her leg is swollen. In the interminable hours of helpless and ignored bystandership in the hospital emergency room, the mother is in a totally different psychological state. Seligman uses this illustration to introduce the two crucial, intimately related concepts of voluntary response and response-outcome independence. There is no question in Seligman's mind that the sense of control is totally related to the freedom of the individual to choose among available alternatives and to perceive the outcome of the dynamic situation as completely contingent on the choice he or she makes.

Thus, in analyzing the housewife's experience at home, Seligman would predict a strong sense of control (or, in Rotter's terms, an internal locus of control). The mother is "a competent parent with a smattering of first aid" who knows the importance of hugs and reassuring words, cleaning the cut, stemming the flow of blood, meanwhile telling the child of her own experience as a little girl and applying antiseptic. Her sense of control is contingent on the outcome of her action, and it is not until her "little girl is happy again and the bleeding has stopped" that she can feel in control. Seligman's point is that in this situation the mother could, at a glance, diagnose and apply appropriate therapy all by herself. By contrast, the hospital situation was one in which "most of [her] actions were to no avail. The hospital staff paid no attention to [her] plight, lost [her] forms, and ignored [her] request for an explanation; [her] child recovered without [her] having brought it about. The course of events was uncontrollable—the outcome was independent of each of [her] voluntary responses."

The crucial issue here is posed by the failure to distinguish between a desirable outcome that is contingent on one's voluntary responses and one that, although not as contingent, nonetheless does not confuse and bewilder one. The latter, too, is consistent with a strong sense of coherence.

Suppose the mother had a positive experience with the emergency room. Suppose the forms had been filled out only after care for the child had been initiated and had not been lost. Suppose the nurse or doctor had come out several times and turned to the mother, keeping her informed, consulting with her, dealing with her as a patient who needed reassurance, and responding to her requests. In other words, suppose everything had happened that was conducive to the mother's feeling that things were under control, that she was part of the picture, though not in control, and that a positive outcome was most likely without there being any need whatsoever for her intervention. Is it not likely that her sense of control would be high?

We can now place control in a historical-cultural context. The writer and most of the readers of this book, as well as Seligman and his suburban mother, have been socialized to mistrust any situation in which we are not personally in control, in which it is not our actions that shape the outcome. Our version of the Protestant Ethic has taught us that we cannot rely on others. In the last analysis, there is no family, no friend, no priest; there is even no God who shows mercy and helps.

This, of course, is the model. In practice, none of us could take the awesome anxiety that would inevitably accompany an existence based on such beliefs. And so we compromise our principles, as it were. Let me make most explicit the two implications of the previous paragraphs. First, I have suggested that even in our most extraordinary culture in its insistence on "my" being in control, in many areas and situations, we are perfectly willing to allocate control to the expert without feeling that our sense of coherence is being violated. The second point is, as it were, a contradiction of the first, yet I believe that both are true. By the very nature of our culture, which leads us to insist so consistently on "my" being in control, we are never comfortable, we remain ambivalent, when we do allocate or when we are compelled to allocate control to others. I shall later consider the implications of this tension and ambivalence in discussing the problem of a fake sense of coherence. For the present, I have been concerned only to point to the distinction, even within our extreme middle-class culture, between being in control over things and things being under control.

This distinction is even more apparent, and the cultural bias more striking, when we turn to a consideration of other cultures. Contrasting these with the dominant value orientation of Western industrial society highlights two issues. First, as suggested above, there is the question of "I am in control" versus "things are under control." Second, there is the issue of the significance of the existence of alternatives and choice. In many societies, the sense of coherence not only is not impaired but is enhanced by the fact that control is located in a deity or in the hands of powerful others. The crucial question is whether, as I have indicated earlier, there is a serene belief that those in control have legitimate power and act in one's own interest. This formulation allows, but does not insist on, the co-identity of the person whose fate is being determined and the decision maker. Think of a Calvinist with a profound belief in predestination. What would someone with a belief that God has already determined his destiny score on Rotter's scale? Familiarity with Calvinist life (or with Christian Science or with orthodox Judaism) suggests the answer to the seeming paradox; I find it in the word *participation*. If life offers one the chance of confirming one's predestined salvation by doing the prescribed right things, one can have a strong sense of coherence. Only when there is no deity, no writ, but only meaningless chaos does one's only hope lie in an internal locus of control. There are, then, many cultural roads to a strong sense of coherence.

The issue of available alternatives as essential to a strong sense of coherence reflects a second aspect of the danger of cultural bias. I have referred to this issue earlier as the danger of overload and hence only make note of it here. As Bensman and Rosenberg have put it (1963, p. 187), "Actual freedom and individual integrity, something often called autonomy or spontaneity, much praised by philosophers and psychologists, have frequently produced a feeling of helplessness." It may be that Americans have been dulled to what for me, having been out of the United States for many years, is still a fresh response to watching television commercials or entering a supermarket; the choices can be so bewildering that they result in a sense of paralysis rather than control. One must add, of course, that in a culture where no deity is potent or relevant, some choice is unquestionably an essential ingredient of a strong sense of coherence.

Having raised the question of cultural—or, as one might put it more sharply, ideological—bias with respect to the locus-of-control approach, I think it only appropriate that the same question be directed at the concept of sense of coherence. Two major inferences might be drawn that could point to such bias. First, a strong sense of coherence could be held to be a good in and of itself. Second, the emphasis on conditions of stability and predictability, whether in childrearing patterns, social structure, or culture, would seem to be inherently conservative. Neither inference is warranted.

I have hypothesized that a strong sense of coherence is salutogenic. Let us assume that the data will support this hypothesis and, further, that health is universally held to be good. Health, however, is only one value. Many in the health professions would have it that it should be the supreme value. This bias leads them to disregard other values or blithely to assume that there is never any conflict between health and other values, that no price is ever paid for doing what is good for one's health. (See Lewis and Lewis,

1977, for an analysis of the implications for health of the growing participation of women in the labor force.) I would make it quite clear. Even if my thesis is supported and a strong sense of coherence is valued because it is good for health, a sense of coherence is still not necessarily praiseworthy as a good in itself. A person with a strong sense of coherence is quite capable of being what many would consider an insensitive, unpleasant, inconsiderate, exploitative bastard. For a good example of what I mean, think of George Bernard Shaw's portrayal of Undershaft in *Major Barbara*. This is precisely one of the reasons why I included the quote from Brinton. In fact, probably the best historical examples of social groups with a strong sense of coherence are ruling classes in their heydays.

The second charge of ideological bias may be seen as even more serious. I have taken the position that social upheaval, rapid social and personal change, and severe conflict may well disrupt a strong sense of coherence. That this position necessarily carries conservative connotations can be refuted on three grounds. First, social conflict is not necessarily disruptive in this sense. It may well provide a firm basis for enhanced rootedness in a subgroup, for strengthened clarity of the meaning of life (see Coser, 1956). Second, so what? Conflict and mobility may be preferred on other grounds even if one pays the price in an impaired sense of coherence. (As a voluntary migrant, I can hardly take any other position.) Third, I would stress that a reasonable degree of repeated experience of challenge and successful resolution strengthens one's sense of coherence. It need not make life incomprehensible, particularly in a society that is tolerant of change, has socialized its members to prefer an ambiance of orderly change and to be tolerant of some ambiguity, and provides the structural conditions for successful resolution of challenge. (See Wertheim, 1974, for consideration of the implied conservatism in the position that autonomy and competence are tied to fitting in neatly into the age, sex, and other slots assigned by one's culture.)

To put the matter even more bluntly. A strong sense of coherence is not compatible with a totalitarian or other type of regime based on terror and naked power (or with analogous personal situations). Nor is it compatible with normless libertarianism, "doing one's own thing." It is, however, quite compatible with a variety of other types of social and personal order: legitimated conservative systems no less than dynamic, democratic consensual systems. There are, to repeat, many sociocultural roads to a strong sense of coherence.

Operationalizing the Sense of Coherence

If the sense of coherence is a concept that seems to have internal and face validity and theoretically offers promise as a powerful research tool, then the next task to be confronted is that of operationalization. Beyond full recognition of the importance of the problem, it would not be appropriate here to explore this issue. Three important points, however, are in order.

First, there is no need—indeed, it would be unfortunate—to commit oneself to a particular methodology. The concept requires much exploration before it can become a systematic tool. Survey questions, a focused interview schedule, observation, use of informants are all in order at this stage of the game. Ultimately, of course, if the concept is to become useful, commitment must be made to a specific operational definition. This can, however, be done prematurely.

Second, I have throughout referred to a strong and a weak sense of coherence. This implied dichotomy, used for the sake of convenience, is misleading. To have written "located toward the strong (or weak) end of the sense-of-coherence continuum" would have been awkward. I hope that the reader has understood that, much as with references to health, I view the concept as referring to a continuum. The researcher who intends using the concept should certainly be aware that it refers to a distribution that is assumed to be normal (bell shaped) rather than bimodal. In this regard, it should be noted that, though Rotter suggested that locus of control refers to a continuum, most studies have dichotomized the scale.

My insistence on a continuum leads us, finally, to consider what I call a fake sense of coherence. A salutogenic orientation, committed to studying those who are indeed toward the strong end of the continuum, is particularly prone to this danger. Lefcourt

(1976, chap. 11) indicates that those who are extremely internal on the locus-of-control scale are prone to paranoia and delusions of grandeur. I would suggest that the core of such fakeness is hysterical rigidity. When there is a contention that all problems have an answer, when challenge or doubt is intolerable, when there is no flexibility to adapt to changing circumstances, when one claims to be in control of all things or to understand everything, when there is a denial of sadness, and when there is an incapacity to admit to the uncontrollable without being overwhelmed—there is a clear indication that we are confronted by a fake sense of coherence.

Chapter Six

Relation of the Sense of Coherence to Health

Up to now we have unavoidably dealt with the issues in piecemeal fashion. Having initially set the problem as that of salutogenesis, we put aside health as the dependent variable so that the concepts of stressor, generalized resistance resources, and the sense of coherence could be clarified. But before the overall salutogenic model can be presented in Chapter Seven, we must consider one crucial question: What are the grounds and evidence for the presumed relationship between location on the sense of coherence continuum and location on the health ease/dis-ease continuum? This continuum was, after all, the point of origin in this endeavor. Asking the salutogenic question has led me to the sense of coherence as a proposed answer. It would take a major research program to test the power of this answer. One can, however, begin to anticipate the results of such a

160

program—or, at least, judge its possible fruitfulness—by considering data now available.

We face two fundamental difficulties in examining the evidence for a relationship between the sense of coherence and health. First, the concept of the sense of coherence has not been operationalized and data have not been assembled that could put the hypothesis to a real test. The data that will be considered were assembled for other purposes. Only by reinterpreting these findings can we consider the possibility that the sense of coherence offers a more adequate or a more parsimonious explanation (or both) than the one offered by previous researchers. Such interpretation is always legitimately suspect. I may be sensitized only to such data as seem to fit my hypothesis and may ignore contradictory data. I can say only that I have not done so consciously, though I make no claim to a mastery of all the data that might be relevant.

The second difficulty arises from the fact that the overwhelming part of the data was assembled with a pathogenic orientation. More particularly and more seriously, almost all but the overall mortality data relate to specific diseases. Seldom do we learn anything about the proportion of a population in a study that is healthy, whatever the definition. For all we know, a higher rate of coronary artery disease in group A than in group B may also be accompanied by a lower rate of cancer in group A.

It seems, then, most sensible to consider the discussion of "evidence" below as no more than an attempt to establish a prima facie case for the plausibility of the hypothesis. I do not wish to sound too diffident. I am persuaded that the sense of coherence is a powerful construct that can be most helpful in understanding a wide variety of data. But it has yet to be tested rigorously.

Somewhat Direct Evidence

In Chapter Five, I referred to the work of Kohn (1968, 1973, 1976a) in which he arrived at an overarching synthesis of the many studies linking social class to schizophrenia. The conditions of life of the lowest social class, he argued, foster limited and rigid conceptions of social reality. This orientation, interacting with powerful stressors and a genetic predisposition, explains the much higher rates of schizophrenia consistently found in the lowest social class. I suggested that a very weak sense of coherence is the precise equivalent of the orientation Kohn described. In a way, however, there is such a great linguistic similarity between the way I have described a weak sense of coherence and the way schizophrenics look at the world that one might well suspect tautology. At best, it might be said that a weak sense of coherence is implicated in schizophrenia but not in other diseases.

The work of Engel and his colleagues, however, is not subject to this charge. Their work on a concept analogous to the sense of coherence, over two decades, led them to conclude (Schmale, 1972, p. 23): "The giving-up process was found as an antecedent to diseases of all categories, from infectious and metabolic to those of degenerative and neoplastic origin in the medical group and from acute organic brain syndromes and schizophrenic reactions to psychoneurotic disorders and the clinical syndromes of depression in the psychiatric group."

But perhaps the most direct support of a link between the sense of coherence and health status is from the study whose data led me to formulate the concept of the sense of coherence (Antonovsky and Shoham, 1978). A sample of 389 Israeli men and women aged forty to forty-nine were selected from the rosters of seven neighborhood health centers in all areas of a middle-sized Israeli city and were interviewed. Some 85 percent of the area population belongs to the health-insurance fund that operates the centers. The dependent variable, health status, is based on an earlier version of, but is essentially similar to, the breakdown continuum presented in Chapter Two. A considerable variety of measures of generalized resistance resources were covered in the largely closed questionnaire: flexibility, self-esteem, a variety of social supports, material resources, and so forth.

One such GRR is of interest here. Deriving it from Engel and Schmale's ideas of helplessness and hopelessness, we called it coping ability. Operationally, four single items and one seven-part item were used.[1] Only when we examined the total structure of the

[1] The items, translated from the Hebrew, are: (1) How often do you run into problems that you think you can't solve? (very often . . . often . . .

data, using a smallest-space analysis, did we realize that we seemed to be dealing with a somewhat different order of phenomenon. Not only were the correlations with the health measure substantially higher than were those between health and other variables, but the data structure suggested to us that coping ability played an intermediary role between a variety of other resources and health. The index based on the seven-part item correlated 0.49 with the measure of health; only the children's needs item showed a correlation of less than 0.40. No other measure in the study had such a high correlation with health except for a life-satisfaction index—that is, what was called, in Chapter Two, other dimensions of well-being.

Indirect Evidence

The studies and data that provide indirect evidence for a relationship between the sense of coherence and health are grouped below in five areas: social-structural, cultural, psychological, situational, and animal studies. In each case, the fundamental argument is the same, namely, that the independent variable provides life experiences related to the level of the sense of coherence and hence to health and illness.

Social-Structural Variables. The literature relating social class to illness is vast. My own work relates to overall mortality and life expectancy, cardiovascular morbidity and mortality, and infant mortality (Antonovsky, 1967a, 1967b, 1968; Antonovsky and Bernstein, 1977). The work on infectious diseases is too well known to be cited. Syme and Berkman (1976), in a succinct review of a wide variety of data, say: "In summary, persons in lower-class

---

occasionally . . . rarely or never). (2) To what extent do you feel that you succeed in solving the problems that you run into? (always or almost always succeed . . . often . . . occasionally . . . never or almost never succeed). (3) Does it happen that you feel that you can't give your children what you would like to give them? (very often . . . often . . . occasionally . . . rarely or never). (4) (Same as item 3 for husband/wife.) (5) During the past few months, have you been in a situation where you felt you were in a trap— that something extremely unpleasant could happen to you or to someone close to you and you were helpless to do anything about it? Did this happen to you (yes or no) with respect to: (a) friends or acquaintances, (b) husband/ wife, (c) children, (d) financial matters, (e) work (or major role activity), (f) your health or that of someone close to you, (g) anything else?

groups have higher morbidity and mortality rates of almost every disease and illness" (p. 2). One needs, then, an overall explanation for such vulnerability to illness in general. They suggest that research be focused on "the more generalized ways in which people deal with problems in their everyday life" (p. 5), an approach clearly consonant with the concept of the sense of coherence. If, then, one premises that a central characteristic of lower-class life is a weak sense of coherence, it seems most reasonable to accept this body of work as suggestive of a relationship between sense of coherence and health status.

Berkman's doctoral dissertation (1977; see also Berkman, in press) is one of the most valuable germane reviews of the literature. Concluding her documented review, she writes (p. 18): "Thus, people who are widows, mobile, or migrants as well as those who are poor or come from certain parts of the country or who are members of certain ethnic groups have higher than expected morbidity or mortality rates from many diseases. . . . One is directed towards the search for some characteristic or set of characteristics which these groups have in common and which in itself has been thought to have deleterious health effects." Berkman proposes that what is common to the poor, blacks, widowers, people who are highly mobile socially or geographically, relocated elderly people, and people with important characteristics different from those of the community in which they live is that they are all subject to powerful socially structured constraints "on an individual's ability to maintain enduring and effective social ties" (p. 19).

Using questionnaire data from a sample of almost 7,000 people aged thirty to sixty-nine, collected in 1965, and the recorded deaths of 682 of the respondents in the following nine-year period, Berkman found strong support for her hypothesis. Her social-network index was found to have a clear association with mortality independent of a wide variety of other risk factors. It would take us too far afield to consider the study in detail, but a number of findings merit note in the present context. Men aged fifty to fifty-nine of lowest socioeconomic status with a high social-network score have a lower mortality rate than do those of highest status with a low network score; women aged thirty to forty-nine in these two polar status/social-network categories have the same lowest mortality rate (pp. 147–148). Though Berkman's theoretical and empirical focus was on those with the lowest social-network score, her data show a linear association—the higher the score, the lower the mortality (pp. 291–292).

In her discussion of what it is about social contacts that may be critical to health, she suggests that social contacts provide tangible support, appraisal support, and emotional support (p. 229). It seems to me reasonable to propose that the concept of a sense of coherence provides a more powerful and parsimonious explanation of differential mortality rates. A strong sense of coherence, on the one hand, is fostered by social supports (and debilitated by migration, being poor, being black in a given society) and, on the other hand, enables one to mobilize tangible, appraisal, and emotional support in coping with stressors.

The same reasoning can be applied to Gove's study (1973) of mortality rates and marital status in the United States from 1959 to 1961. He clearly shows that the "mortality rates of the unmarried . . . are, controlling for age, higher than those of the married, and the differences between the married and unmarried . . . are much greater for men than for women" (p. 61). The variations are particularly large "where one's psychological state (1) appears to play a direct role in death, as with suicide, homicide, and accidents, (2) is directly related to acts such as alcoholism that frequently lead to death, and (3) would appear to affect one's willingness and ability to undergo the drawn-out and careful treatment required" (p. 61). If being married, then, provides protection, particularly for men, is it not possible that this structural variable facilitates a strong sense of coherence?

Perhaps the most intriguing indirect evidence linking the sense of coherence to health status via social-structural variables is found in the phenomenon of voodoo death. Seligman's section on death from helplessness in humans (1975, pp. 175–188) reviews reports ranging from Cannon's examples of hex death to the death rate of American prisoners of war in the Philippine campaign of World War II. Common to all cases is a social situation in which the person is traumatically stripped of social identity and in which his or her expectations of stability are dramatically destroyed. A nonperson, Seligman suggests, cannot remain alive, particularly

when the social structure that gives validity to existence predicts his
or her demise.

A high degree of status integration—occupancy of social
roles that set compatible norms—may also be conducive to a
strong sense of coherence. In a study subject to methodological criticism but pertinent to our present topic, Dodge and Martin (1970)
review a considerable body of evidence relating status integration to
what they call stress diseases. Their focus is ecological rather than
individual. Of the 136 correlation coefficients on rates of chronic-
disease mortality and status integration, 89 percent were negative
as predicted.

A review of the literature on the particular social-structural
changes involved in bereavement led Jacobs and Ostfeld (1977,
p. 344) to conclude that "the attributable risk of mortality in persons suffering a conjugal bereavement . . . may be as high as 50
percent." They apply Parkes' concept of psychosocial transitions
(1971) in analyzing this phenomenon and link it to Engel and
Schmale's (1972) conservation-withdrawal reaction. In the eight
studies covered, "a basic pattern of excess mortality in the widowed,
especially in males, is discernible. . . . The duration of the elevated risk . . . is no more than two years" (p. 349). The two
qualifications of the overall findings are particularly germane. The
sense of coherence of widows in Western cultures, I suggest, is less
vulnerable to the death of a spouse than is that of widowers. Further, if one does indeed survive the traumatic impact on one's sense
of coherence, it is likely that recovery to the previous level can take
place in a relatively short time.

We now turn, in this review of social-structural factors, to
the work of the late John Cassel and his associates (Cassel, 1974,
1976; Kaplan, Cassel, and Gore, 1977; Nuckolls, Cassel, and
Kaplan, 1972). "A remarkably similar set of social circumstances,"
Cassel writes, "characterizes people who develop tuberculosis and
schizophrenia, alcoholics, victims of multiple accidents, and suicides.
Common to all these people is a marginal status in society. They
are individuals who for a variety of reasons . . . have been de-
prived of meaningful social contact" (1974, p. 474). He later
speaks of "disordered relationships, . . . this failure of various

forms of behavior to elicit predictable responses. . . . These behavioral acts are in a sense inappropriate. . . . The actor is not receiving adequate evidence [feedback] that his actions are leading to anticipated consequences" (pp. 476–477). These notions, derived from animal studies (see below), are then applied by Cassel to suggest an explanation of elevated blood-pressure levels among Zulu urban migrants, of Syme's work on coronary heart disease among migrants, of his own studies on heart disease in counties varying according to degree of urbanization and the health status of first- and second-generation factory workers, as well as of work on mental disorders and stroke.

In a study summarized by Cassel and detailed in Nuckolls, Cassel, and Kaplan (1972, p. 438), "the adaptive potential for pregnancy score" was used to measure psychosocial assets. The fascinating result of this study, for present purposes, is that "in the presence of mounting life change . . . women with high psychosocial assets had only one third the complication rate of women whose psychosocial assets were low." To transpose into my terms: Given a high level of stressors, which leads to tension, a strong sense of coherence (psychosocial assets, social supports) acts to prevent complications in pregnancy. In my own recalculation of the data, there is even a hint that being high on stressors, given high social supports, is salutary. This interpretation would fit the salutogenic hypothesis even more neatly.

The Kaplan, Cassel, and Gore (1977) paper is an attempt of the Cassel group to clarify the social-support hypothesis and review the literature, showing its consequences for biomedical events. They conceive of a stressor situation as involving "the inability of the individual to obtain meaningful information that his actions are leading to desired consequences." Protective factors—for example, social supports—are seen as interacting with stressors to "determine to a considerable extent the susceptibility of the organism to physicochemical disease agents" (p. 18). A creative and extremely useful analysis of social supports follows. But the authors unfortunately stop short of putting the question that begs to be asked: Why are social supports related to health status? They have almost given the answer in characterizing stressors: Social supports enhance the ability of the individual to obtain meaningful information, or, in my terms, enhance the sense of coherence. (For an additional review of the social-support literature, see Cobb, 1976.)

A final study to be noted here is a review by Kiritz and Moos (1974) of "dimensions of the social environment." Though most of their citations refer to short-term physiological changes, they do include a number of studies of morbidity—for example, growth retardation and susceptibility to disease in infants, hypertension, peptic ulcer, coronary heart disease, and rheumatoid arthritis, as well as deaths among older persons. For present purposes, what is most relevant is their systematic conceptualization of three basic types of dimensions that characterize social climates: relationship dimensions—involvement, affiliation, peer cohesion, expressiveness; personal-development dimensions—autonomy, a practical orientation, responsibility; and system-maintenance and system-change dimensions—order, clarity, control, work pressure, innovation. Under these headings, the authors review studies that show how a given social environment, characterized by being high or low on these dimensions, relates to certain health outcomes. Again and again, one is struck by the ease with which one can translate these dimensions into the overarching framework provided by the concept of the sense of coherence. Thus, for example, they cite a study of air-traffic controllers who, working under conditions of heavy responsibility and extreme time pressure, show higher risk and earlier onset of hypertension and peptic ulcer than do those in a control group (Cobb and Rose, 1973). This finding, in my view, relates almost directly to the sense of coherence: the constant bombardment by stimuli in a situation fraught with trepidation that they cannot be handled coherently and fraught with knowledge of the possibility of disastrous consequences.

Cultural Variables. There is considerable overlap between social-structural and cultural variables. A number of the studies mentioned above (Berkman, Dodge and Martin, Cassel) do not find it necessary to distinguish between locations in a social structure that impair the sense of coherence of their occupants and locations in a cultural milieu that act in the same direction. Indeed, the distinction is largely analytical. But it may be useful to briefly take note of a number of additional studies that focus directly on cultural variables.

We turn first to those studies that consider the urban environment, which is most aptly characterized as a cultural pattern of information-input overload. While most of the work that is not largely speculative is based on laboratory animal studies or does not indicate clear pathology as a dependent variable, some results do point to the relationship between noise, crowding, and so forth and essential hypertension. The crucial variable to be studied is, as Ostfeld and D'Atri (1975) put it, "an inability to structure one's social and physical environment" in an urban culture. That it is indeed the sociopsychological rather than the physical factors of the urban environment that are crucial to health status is convincingly demonstrated in a major collaborative effort (Hinkle and Loring, 1977, particularly the papers by Hinkle and by Kasl). Reviewing several hundred studies, Kasl does not accept the oversimplified notion that "there is no evidence of any direct effects of the residential environment on health." Despite some evidence of such direct effects, he suggests that a more powerful model of the complex relationship between environment and health should use "the notion of a person-environment fit" as "the integrating concept" (1977, p. 108).

More direct evidence on the relationship between morbidity and cultural incongruity, or cultural transition or change, or however it is variously termed by different authors—all clearly related to the sense of coherence—is found in Wolff's edited work (Wolf and Goodell, 1968). The editors write of American Indian tribes "taken from their home land and put into reservations within a few miles' distance, in essentially the same physical environment, but in a setting of social disorganization, with a resultant appalling increase in mortality from tuberculosis" (p. 8). A similar result is reported for Bantu natives who had been moved from the countryside outside of Johannesburg into the environs of the city (p. 193). As a third example of morbidity and mortality associated with a radical change in physical and social environment, they cite the study of epidemics of meningococcus meningitis that occurred with the onset of barrack life in the U.S. Army (p. 193).

Most pertinent of all is their summary of the widely known
study of 100 Chinese expatriates in New York. With detailed information on health histories, Hinkle and Wolff (1957) were
able to distinguish between those who were consistently healthy
and those who were, with a substantial degree of consistency, ill.
Wolf and Goodell summarize the study (pp. 204–205): "They
had shared a life in which they had all been exposed to a rapidly
changing culture, repeated disruptions of old social patterns, and
many physical dislocations. . . . The healthiest members of this
group are people who are able to tolerate with some ease such
recurrent disruptions of their life patterns, partly because they regard such changes and disruptions as a normal and expected part
of a life pattern. . . . Hinkle and Wolff infer that ill health . . .
appears to occur when an individual exists in a life situation which
places demands upon him that are excessive in terms of his ability
to meet them."

It seems reasonable to view these findings as corroborating
the hypothesis that when people, for whatever reason, are somehow
able to translate a difficult, complex bombardment of stimuli into
a whole that is meaningful, high health levels are likely to be
maintained. Thus, while there is little doubt that the evidence
points to cultural disruption and transition, which involve a weakening of the sense of coherence, as dysfunctional for health, some
people are capable in these circumstances of maintaining a sense
of coherence. The crucial GRR in such cases, I would suggest, is
what I have called a rational, flexible, and farsighted coping
strategy.

In the major summary of the pertinent studies done in
Hinkle and Wolff's Cornell Human Ecology Study Program—a
summary that reviews some of the above studies as well as those
of American telephone workers, managers, Hungarian refugees,
and others—Hinkle (1974) writes in conclusion: "If a culture
change, social change, or change in interpersonal relations is not
associated with a significant change in the activities, habits, in-
gestants, exposure to disease-causing agents, or in the physical
characteristics of the environment of a person, then its effect upon
his health cannot be defined solely by its nature, its magnitude,
its acuteness or chronicity, or its apparent importance in the eyes

of others" (p. 42). Yet Hinkle has studied many people who have undergone such changes without becoming ill. His key explanation is that certain "psychological characteristics . . . help to 'insulate' them from the effects of some of their life experiences" (p. 40). The core of such psychological characteristics, I would suggest, is a strong sense of coherence.

In the early 1960s, Cassel's team conducted a number of studies of first- and second-generation factory workers and of residents in areas undergoing rapid urbanization and industrialization (Cassel, Patrick, and Jenkins, 1960; Cassel and Tyroler, 1961; Tyroler and Cassel, 1964). On the basis of their findings, they provided one of the earliest formulations of the cultural-disorganization hypothesis, totally consonant with the construct of the sense of coherence. They write, "Rapid culture change is likely to have deleterious health consequences when it leads to the development of incongruities between the culture of the population at risk and the demands and expectations of the new social situation" (Tyroler and Cassel, 1964, p. 167). Unfortunately, this proposal seems to have been too daring to them, for in closing their paper they retreat to an explanation somewhat more palatable to the medical model and focus on "deleterious changes accompanying urbanization . . . [such as] diet, level of physical activity, cigarette smoking, and meeting of deadlines" (p. 175). Not until a decade later (Cassel, 1974) was Cassel to develop his earlier, most important insight.

As a final note in this section, I would mention one of the first works in the field. In a study of enlisted American naval personnel and civilians, Ruesch (1948, p. 91) found that "among ulcer bearers there is an unusual frequency of individuals in the process of culture change. . . . The results indicate that acculturation and social mobility are one of the most important sources of stress among ulcer bearers."

Psychological Variables. Since Rotter (1966) published his work on the locus-of-control concept, a considerable amount of research done on this psychological construct (admirably summarized by Lefcourt, 1976) has been closely related to the sense of coherence. For the most part, however, the studies have focused on the consequences of the locus of control for problem solving and other performance measures and for physiological parameters, and they have been conducted in experimental laboratory situations. The focus on more direct measures of health has been limited to animal studies (see below).

Not until the publication of Seligman's book (1975) was the attempt made to establish a clear link between external locus of control—or, in Seligman's terms, learned helplessness—and the clinical entity of depression. I consider Seligman's work in Chapter Five, where I try to show its close relationship to the sense of coherence. I mention it again here in order to refer to Seligman's chap. 5, which is devoted to analyzing the relationship between learned helplessness and depression. Though providing no hard evidence, he does provide a careful, systematic analysis of six characteristics common to the two variables; this commonality provides reasonable evidence that the two variables are indeed related. In this regard, and as a way of linking social-structural variables to depression, note should be taken of Pearlin and Johnson's work. Their review of relevant studies (1977; see also Pearlin, 1975) proposes a link between "durable, structured conditions of life" (of unmarried people) and depression; Seligman's hypothesis might well be understood within this context.

Frank (1975) stresses the centrality of the "patients' own healing powers" in "the restoration of healthy equilibrium." Despite the fact that he clearly operates within the healthy-sick dichotomous model and both as clinician and theoretician is concerned primarily with restoration, his exploration of the issue of "expectant faith" takes us one step beyond the amorphous will-to-live concept. In addition to some of the studies mentioned above, Frank reports others that have a direct bearing on the sense of coherence and its relationship to health. Thus, for example, he writes of the failure of a group of soldiers with schistosomiasis to recover as expected. Interviewed, they were characterized as having a "destructive mental state"; ambiguity, a feeling that nobody was concerned about their welfare, a lack of authoritative information, alarmist rumors, and a perceived serious threat to survival were the sources of their state of mind.

Other studies cited by Frank refer to information provided before tonsillectomies, recovery from brucellosis and influenza, and speed of healing of a detached retina. In all, Frank sees the psy-

chological state of the patient as intimately and causally related
to recovery. A patient with a high level of expectant faith is a
promising patient. His analysis goes on to consider the miracle
cures of faith healers and placebos, but for our purposes his interpretation of the data is crucial. The physician, he writes, is able
to facilitate the desired state of expectant faith in the patient
because (my emphasis) "he mobilizes in the patient the attitudes
of trust and dependency that a child feels toward a good parent.
. . . His treatment is validated by a theory which both expresses
and *confirms the world view* of the society in which both he and
the patient function. . . . A *shared world view both makes sense
out of life and reinforces the sense of group belongingness*" (p. 52).
I have extremely serious reservations both about Frank's assumptions, indicated in this quote, about the reality of the patient-
doctor relationship and about the extremely manipulative approach
he suggests throughout his paper. These issues I explore in Chapter
Eight. For present purposes, it seems reasonable to infer that the
work reviewed by Frank has a clear affinity to the concept of the
sense of coherence.

Frank also goes on to cite the controversial work of Bahnson and Leshan with regard to cancer patients. Leshan's work
(1978; for a scathing review, see Medawar, 1977) can hardly
be cited as scientific evidence of the causal role psychological factors
may play in cancer, but it is germane because of his theoretical
approach. A psychotherapist, he reports on working with some
seventy cancer patients. He was repeatedly struck by a loss in these
patients of a reason for existing, which followed a loss of a relationship of deep meaning (compare with Engel's concept of giving-up),
and by an absence of direction or goal. "They felt," he writes, "a
lack of any stable reference points for themselves in the universe,
. . . a sense of loneliness and unrelatedness." This world view, he
argues, antedates the illness. Both Leshan and Bahnson (1966,
1974) propose that cancer patients, more than controls, manifest
a personality style of repressing or denying unpleasant affects such
as depression, anxiety, and hostility.

Probably the most exciting and certainly the best known
work that bears a close relationship to the concept of the sense of
coherence is Ray Rosenman and Meyer Friedman's development

of the relationship between coronary heart disease and the Type A behavior pattern. (For present purposes, I have thought it adequate to cite, from the extensive literature, only the paper by Mathews and others, 1977.) Serious evidence shows that individuals who are "competitive, achievement oriented, involved in multiple activities with deadlines, . . . impatient with slowness in others, [and who] like to set a rapid work pace and tend to be hostile and aggressive" have higher prevalence and incidence rates of coronary heart disease (p. 489). In an attempt to identify the crucial elements in the rather global Type A pattern, a detailed study was conducted of 62 coronary cases and 124 coronary disease–free controls. All were selected from a large-scale prospective study conducted in California in 1960–1961. The data were collected when all respondents were coronary disease–free. On the basis of the original interview, each respondent was classified as having given a Type A or Type B response on thirty-seven content items, three speech-stylistic items, and four clinical-judgment items. Factor analysis revealed these forty-four items to cluster in five scores: competitive drive, past achievements, impatience, nonjob achievement, and speed. Only competitive drive and impatience scores were found to be significantly higher among patients than among controls.

I have gone into detail in reporting this study because it is, for the time being, the culmination of a large body of serious work on the major chronic disease facing Western societies. The crucial question I would pose is: What is it about the Type A behavior pattern that explains its association with coronary heart disease over and above the more conventional risk factors (smoking, hypertension, cholesterol)? We would do best to consider the discussion by Mathews and others (my emphasis): "A high drive level, coupled with impatience and hostility, is readily apparent in the characteristic tendency of Type As to seek ever-expanding goals and achievements. . . . They have tried to change but have reverted to their hard-driving activities as they found themselves becoming increasingly anxious about work which still needed to be finished and goals that had not yet been attained. . . . *Impending lack of control is experienced as anxiety arousing.* . . . Pattern A may indeed be interpreted as a response style for coping with threats to a sense of environmental mastery and control" (p. 496).

Unfortunately, the authors do not explicitly take the final step that would make their description of the Type A pattern almost a perfect equivalent of a weak sense of coherence. The step just begs to be taken by their own words. It is not just the competitive drive and impatience that matter. The two together, and consideration of the specific items that make up these factor scores, point to an underlying global orientation that leads one to expect that no matter how hard one tries life is so organized that one will never succeed in its being under control. One of the authors, writing elsewhere (Glass, 1977), indeed concurs with this interpretation: "Type As are engaged in a struggle for control. . . . Pattern A behavior is a strategy for coping with uncontrollable stress; enhanced performance reflects an attempt to assert and maintain control after its loss has been threatened" (pp. 181–182).

In this paper, Glass also touches on an issue that is most salient here. He makes the necessary distinction between Type A as a behavior pattern and as a global orientation of learned helplessness (a weak sense of coherence), a concept he takes from Seligman. He suggests that Type A behavior, following "extended experience with salient uncontrollable stress, results in enhanced vulnerability to helplessness among Type As" (p. 184), and hence it is a precursor to coronary disease. We do not have evidence that Type As are less vulnerable to other diseases. But even if this should prove to be the case, it would not contradict the hypothesis that a weak sense of coherence is crucial to dis-ease. Quite the contrary may be true. In other words, a weak sense of coherence combined with Type A behavior and failure to maintain environmental control (combined with other variables, genetic, constitutional, environmental, and behavioral) may lead to coronary heart disease. A weak sense of coherence combined with other variables may lead to cancer, and so on. The salutogenic orientation, as I have repeatedly stressed, compels us to search for themes common to health ease, rather than factors in specific diseases.

Situational Variables. We now turn to the fourth major category of studies that may be seen to provide indirect evidence for the existence of a relationship between a strong sense of coherence and health. Because the literature is vast, I limit myself to the one volume that is the most valuable concentration of work in the area, the proceedings of a conference on stressful life events organized by Barbara and Bruce Dohrenwend in 1973 (1974; see also Gunderson and Rahe, 1974).

The concern with life events as possible factors in the etiology of various somatic and psychological disorders in this century can be traced to W. B. Cannon and Adolph Meyer. For present purposes, I confine my discussion to what has become the major school in this area rather than consider life events as equivalent with all stressors. The Holmes-Rahe Social Readjustment Rating Scale and the Schedule of Recent Experiences have been the most widely used instruments in this school. As Holmes and Masuda (1974) describe the development of the forty-three-item rating scale, it originated in the Cornell Human Ecology Study Program when investigators studying the protocols of thousands of patients were struck by repeated reporting of life events "whose advent is either indicative of, or requires a significant change in, the ongoing life pattern of the individual. The emphasis is on change from the existing steady state and not on psychological meaning, emotion, or social desirability" (p. 46). Holmes and his colleagues were persuaded "that a cluster of social events that require change in ongoing life adjustment is significantly associated with the time of illness onset" (p. 47). They turned to devising a weighting scale for each of the forty-three items, based on a broad degree of consensus in a considerable number of populations, both American and non-American. Thus death of a spouse is scored 100, marriage, 50, and minor violations of the law, 11.

Before the final development of this instrument, retrospective studies using the same approach had shown that "life events cluster significantly in the two-year period preceding onset of tuberculosis, heart disease, skin disease, hernia, and pregnancy" (p. 57). Later studies have shown relationships between life change scores and sudden cardiac death, time of onset of myocardial infarction, and fractures. Subsequently, work began on prospective studies, the best known of which is Rahe's study of U.S. Navy personnel aboard three cruisers at sea for six months; he found that life change scores could predict reported illness. Holmes and Masuda conclude their review of the data by saying (p. 67), "The greater the life change or adaptive requirement, the greater the vulnerability or lowering of resistance to disease, and the more serious the disease that does develop. . . . Thus, the concept of life change appears to have relevance to the causation of disease, time of onset of disease, and severity of disease. It does not seem to contribute much to an understanding of specificity of disease type."

Holmes has insisted that this approach was derived empirically and has worked consistently. Rahe (1974) has sought to develop a more sophisticated theoretical understanding of why one should expect to find a relationship between life change scores and illness. He proposes a chain of events involving life changes, psychological defenses that filter out some changes as nonsignificant, physiological reactions to those events not filtered out, coping—attempting to reduce physiological reactions, illness behavior, and identified illness.

There are clearly many serious methodological problems, and much more research is required before any firm conclusion is possible about the life-events approach. The Dohrenwend volume raises most of these problems and includes findings that stress the negative life events, or events involving exits from social relationships, as being important in facilitating illness. If indeed it should prove to be the case that negative life events are critical to breakdown, I suggest such a connection would be consistent with the sense-of-coherence approach. Rahe's theoretical position suggests this relationship. The adult with a strong sense of coherence is, if my analysis has been correct, certainly capable of mobilizing resources to cope with the adaptive demands of life changes, whether positive or negative. The person with a weak sense of coherence meets the adaptive requirement with a sense of helplessness, which becomes a self-fulfilling prophecy; he or she sees the life change as not making sense and therefore is incapable of successful adaptation.

It may be that Holmes' original position will prove to be correct—that is, that life change scores per se are decisive for health and illness, irrespective of whether people have a strong or weak sense of coherence. My own position is unquestionably different. There is, of course, a relationship between life events and the sense of coherence, which I spell out in Chapter Seven. But, I would hypothesize, given the same life-events score, people with different strengths of the sense of coherence manifest different health outcomes. And, conversely, I anticipate that people with the same level of the sense of coherence but different life-events scores are equally healthy. As a matter of fact, as suggested earlier, I would not even be surprised if a moderately high life-events score that does not shake up the sense of coherence turns out to be salutary.

The life-events data, then, constitute one set of evidence that does not support the sense of coherence thesis. As Rahe's recent work suggests, however, there may not be as much of a contradiction between the two approaches as first seems to be apparent. In any case, I believe there is good reason to support considerable research to test the alternative approaches.

A series of studies have dealt with one life situation that, if anything, involves stability rather than change and has long been presumed to be related to health. Crowding—in the sense of both persons per room and density in a geographical area—has in itself, over and above other factors associated with it, like poverty, been implicated as an etiological factor. The common sense hypothesis, based on considerable evidence that failed to separate out crowding per se from other variables as a cause of infectious diseases, merits closer analysis.

In one review of the evidence, Cassel (1977) casts considerable doubt on the presumed relationship between crowding and even infectious diseases. As he reads the evidence, the crucial variable is not at all any measure of density but rather "the pattern of relationship that exists" among the people being studied. Disordered relationships, he suggests, are crucial to morbid consequences. They "often have in common a failure to elicit anticipated responses to what were previously appropriate cues and an increasing disregard of traditional obligations and rights" (p. 133). Cassel goes on to hypothesize: "In human populations, increased susceptibility to disease should occur when, for a variety of reasons, individuals do not receive any evidence [feedback] that their actions are leading to desirable and anticipated consequences" (p. 133). In other words, as the most recent evidence on crowding, including studies in Hong Kong, Holland, and Canada (Booth and Cowell, 1976), suggests, when a high degree of crowding is accompanied by social and interpersonal disorganization, there will be deleterious consequences for health. The compatibility between Cassel's words and the concept of the sense of coherence should be noted. In all justice, I should make it explicit that Cassel's work and his words have been a direct and influential factor in my development of the concept.

Animal Studies. I do not hold much of a brief for using laboratory studies of animals as evidence for a relationship between the sense of coherence and health. Handled carefully, however, a consistent pattern of results can give rise to fruitful hypotheses about people. This is indeed the approach Cassel has used (1974, 1977). An early study with a unique twist—the idea for the study is attributed to Spitz' work on maternal deprivation—is reported by Liddell (1954). His experimental procedures were quite successful in showing how "psychological stress" can lead to neurotic behavior and death in sheep and goats. The same stress introduced in the presence of the animal's mother, however, brought no adverse consequences. Cassel (1974) and Seligman (1975) both review the experimental evidence, all of which seems to indicate that it is the social conditions under which stressors—electric shock, insoluble problems, crowding, deprivation—are imposed that are decisive in health outcomes. Unfortunately, these experiments have all focused on pathogenic outcomes, with much less careful manipulation of the variables that might be decisive in salutogenic outcomes.

Engel (1974), it seems to me, has come closest to formulating an interpretation of many animal studies. Cleverly, he "asked" rats, as a good clinician would do, when they develop ulcers. The answer he was "given" is interpreted in accord with the giving-up hypothesis. Engel's words, however, are almost closer to the concept of the sense of coherence than to his own formulation: "the immobilized rat [was unable] to do anything about his situation. . . . The most effective protection against ulcerogenesis was afforded by devising situations in which the animal received reliable feedback information that what it was doing was the right thing to avoid shock. . . . The organism [lost its ability] to predict and maintain control over its environment" (p. 1090).

I have reviewed a considerable number of empirical studies relating psychosocial factors to health outcomes. With few exceptions, the results of these studies are at least compatible with hypotheses that would be derived from the concept of the sense of coherence. This compatibility suggests that there are serious grounds for a large-scale empirical program of research. Yet I would go much further. I propose that this construct is not just another variable to be studied. It is, rather, a most parsimonious way of subsuming a great variety of discrete variables, from mother's presence through work overload-underload balance to information provided to patients.

But two further clarifications—or, rather, reiterations—are required. First, I have explicitly committed myself to the thesis that the concept of a sense of coherence is a global orientation that is pervasive and enduring. My contention has been that fluctuations over relatively limited periods of time or in different situations are relatively minor (barring traumatic experiences; see Chapter Seven). This contention must, of course, be put to the test. The methodological implications are considerable as far as populations, situations, and tools of measurement are concerned.

Second, I have intentionally made no mention of the mechanisms and channels through which the sense of coherence is related to health. Not only is this question outside the scope of my professional competence, but a number of workers in the field have written quite plausible postulates concerning the all-important link. The reader concerned with this question might do well to look at the work (going beyond Selye, of course) of Cassel (1974), Glass (1977), Kagan and Levi (1974), and Levi (1974). In considering this work, I would point up one distinction that, as I indicated in Chapter Three, seems to me to be crucial—the fundamental distinction between a state of tension and a state of stress. Not all those who analyze the stress responses of organisms to psychosocial stressors —or, in my terms, the response of people to living in general, whatever the strength of the sense of coherence—are sensitive to the difference. Kagan and Levi come fairly close (p. 227): "It has been claimed that if a sympatho-adrenomedullary stimulation lasts too long or is repeated too often, the result will first be unpleasant functional disturbances in various organs and organ systems. . . . Such a dysfunction, if long standing and/or intense, may result in permanent structural changes of pathogenic significance at least in predisposed individuals."

The work, however, that seems to me to be most congenial to the salutogenic approach is that of Solomon and Amkraut (1974). True, they initially state that "stress and emotional distress may influence the function of the immunologic system via central nervous system disease and endocrine mediation." Their concept of immunological balance, however, opens up the way for the study of how a strong sense of coherence may be linked to maintaining one's location on or moving toward the ease end of the health ease/disease continuum. It may be that when confronted with stressors, the person with a strong sense of coherence can activate a variety of immunological factors, thereby preventing tension from being transformed into stress.

I have now completed the inevitably partial discussion of each segment of the salutogenic model. The time has come to put all the pieces together. For this, we turn to Chapter Seven.

Chapter Seven

The Salutogenic
Model of Health

In Chapter One, I posed the problem of salutogenesis. Chapter Two proposed a solution to the problem of the measurement of health status consonant with the salutogenic orientation. At that point, the core of the question was put as the need to explain the location of a person near the ease end of the health ease/dis-ease continuum. Chapter Three considered—and rejected—the hypothesis that the answer could be stressor avoidance. In Chapter Four, an initial alternative answer was presented: the availability of generalized resistance resources. The initial question was also broadened to consider maintenance or improvement of one's position on the breakdown continuum, irrespective of location at any given time. Analysis of the nature of generalized resistance resources, of why they are hypothesized to facilitate tension management and avoid stress, led to the formulation of the central construct of the book, the sense of coherence, considered at length in Chapter Five. The final building block in what I call the salutogenic model appears in Chapter Six, which presents the evidence for linking the sense of coherence and health status.

Inevitably, detailed consideration of each building block obscures the integral character of the model as a whole. Paradoxically, further, it oversimplifies a complex of interrelationships. Finally, it tends to obscure the links between the variables in the model. The function of this chapter, then, is to overcome these difficulties. The full picture, as I see it, is presented in Figure 1. A model frozen in a diagram unfortunately has a static character. It takes a leap of the imagination to transform both the elements in the model and the arrows and lines indicating their interrelationships into a dynamic whole in space and particularly in time. But the diagram is the best I can do, and I would ask the reader to refer to it as each element and link is discussed.

Sense of Coherence

Studying a diagram or discussing it in words requires an element of arbitrariness in selecting a point of departure. It is nonetheless not accidental that I start the discussion from the sense of coherence. This is, after all, the core of my answer to the problem of salutogenesis. The sense of coherence is measurable; each of us is located at some point on the sense-of-coherence continuum, which can be seen as an ordinal scale. Sense of coherence is an orientation that is not situation- or role-specific. Although there may be situations or issues with regard to which a person with a strong sense of coherence can be utterly perplexed, these are essentially peripheral to one's life or mark minor fluctuations around a fairly stable location on the continuum. Given the nature of human existence, it is difficult to conceive of anyone being extremely high on the continuum. This would require an unimaginably stable world, an inconceivably unchanging internal and external environment. Only someone who is totally out of touch with reality could claim to have an absolute sense of coherence. In fact, in Chapter Five I suggest that a good clue to a fake sense of coherence would be an extremely high score. Most of us, then, would score from extremely low to moderately high.

Figure 1
The Salutogenic Model

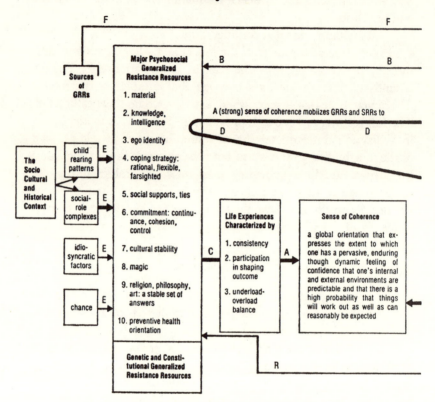

Key to Figure 1

Arrow A: **Life experiences shape the sense of coherence.**

Arrow B: Stressors affect the generalized resistance resources at one's disposal.

Line C: **By definition, a GRR provides one with sets of meaningful, coherent life experiences.**

Arrow D: **A strong sense of coherence mobilizes the GRRs and SRRs at one's disposal.**

Arrows E: **Childrearing patterns, social role complexes,** idiosyncratic factors, and chance build up GRRs.

Arrow F: The sources of GRRs also create stressors.

Arrow G: Traumatic physical and biochemical stressors affect health status directly; health status affects extent of exposure to psychosocial stressors.

Arrow H: Physical and biochemical stressors interact with endogenic pathogens and "weak links" and with stress to affect health status.

Arrow I: Public and private health measures avoid or neutralize stressors.

Line J: A strong sense of coherence, mobilizing GRRs and SRRs, avoids stressors.

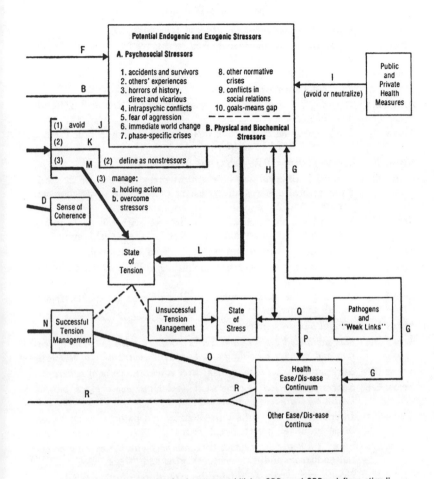

Line K: A strong sense of coherence, mobilizing GRRs and SRRs, defines stimuli as nonstressors.

Arrow L: **Ubiquitous stressors create a state of tension.**

Arrow M: **The mobilized GRRs (and SRRs) interact with the state of tension and manage a holding action and the overcoming of stressors.**

Arrow N: **Successful tension management strengthens the sense of coherence.**

Arrow O: **Successful tension management maintains one's place on the health ease/dis-ease continuum.**

Arrow P: Interaction between the state of stress and pathogens and "weak links" negatively affects health status.

Arrow Q: Stress is a general precursor that interacts with the existing potential endogenous and exogenous pathogens and "weak links."

Arrow R: Good health status facilitates the acquisition of other GRRs.

Note: The statements in bold type represent the core of the salutogenic model.

Key to Figure 1

Arrow A: *Life experiences shape the sense of coherence.*

Arrow B: Stressors affect the generalized resistance resources at one's disposal.

Line C: *By definition, a GRR provides one with sets of meaningful, coherent life experiences.*

Arrow D: *A strong sense of coherence mobilizes the GRRs and SRRs at one's disposal.*

Arrows E: *Childrearing patterns, social role complexes,* idiosyncratic factors, and chance *build up GRRs.*

Arrow F: The sources of GRRs also create stressors.

Arrow G: Traumatic physical and biochemical stressors affect health status directly; health status affects extent of exposure to psychosocial stressors.

Arrow H: Physical and biochemical stressors interact with endogenic pathogens and "weak links" and with stress to affect health status.

Arrow I: Public and private health measures avoid or neutralize stressors.

Line J: A strong sense of coherence, mobilizing GRRs and SRRs, avoids stressors.

Line K: A strong sense of coherence, mobilizing GRRs and SRRs, defines stimuli as nonstressors.

Arrow L: *Ubiquitous stressors create a state of tension.*

Arrow M: *The mobilized GRRs (and SRRs) interact with the state of tension and manage a holding action and the overcoming of stressors.*

Arrow N: *Successful tension management strengthens the sense of coherence.*

Arrow O: *Successful tension management maintains one's place on the health ease/dis-ease continuum.*

Arrow P: Interaction between the state of stress and pathogens and "weak links" negatively affects health status.

Arrow Q: Stress is a general precursor that interacts with the existing potential endogenic and exogenic pathogens and "weak links."

Arrow R: Good health status facilitates the acquisition of other GRRs.

Note: The statements in italic type are the core of the salutogenic model.

To say that the sense of coherence is stable, enduring, and pervasive does not, however, compel us to say that it is immutable. In what sense, then, is it dynamic? We would do well to divide the answer to this question into two parts. The first focuses on the development of the orientation in childhood, adolescence, and early adulthood. The second considers modifications throughout subsequent life. The two parts overlap: there can be sharp changes of direction in childhood; there is development throughout life until death. But it is analytically useful to deal separately with the emergence of a sense of coherence and then with its modification.

Life Experiences

As indicated in the diagram, life experiences (Arrow A) are crucial in shaping a sense of coherence. From the time of birth, or even earlier, we constantly go through situations of challenge and response, stress, tension, and resolution. The more these experiences are characterized by consistency, participation in shaping outcome, and an underload-overload balance of stimuli, the more we begin to see the world as being coherent and predictable. When, however, one's experiences all tend to be predictable, one is inevitably due for unpleasant surprises that cannot be handled, and one's sense of coherence is weakened accordingly. Paradoxically, then, a measure of unpredictable experiences—which call forth hitherto unknown resources—is essential for a strong sense of coherence. One then learns to expect some measure of the unexpected. When there is little or no predictability, there is not much one can do except seek to hide until the storm (of life) is over, hoping not to be noticed. Or else one strikes out blindly and at random until exhaustion sets in. No defense mechanisms can be adequate.

We must note an implicit assumption here. If a strong sense of coherence is to develop, one's experiences must be not only by and large predictable but also by and large rewarding, yet with some measure of frustration and punishment. The outcome depends on the underload-overload balance. But what if one's life experiences are largely consistent and predictable but frustrating and punishing? Again, the answer is a matter of degree. Frustration and punishment can be so devastating that survival is put into question. If they are not so extreme, then defense mechanisms become possible and a reasonably strong sense of coherence begins to form.

One emerges from childhood, then, with some formed albeit tentative sense of coherence. In adolescence, the crucial stage for ego identity, tentativeness begins to be transformed into definitiveness. If one's experiences continue to be by and large cut of the same cloth as earlier experiences, one's sense of coherence is reinforced.

Yet considerable change is possible. The important point is that there is increasing room for choice. The child maintains a small number of salient relationships. He gets feedback from relatively few people. The stimuli are not too variable. The adolescent has greater options in choosing or encountering experiences that enhance or weaken his or her sense of coherence.

Entering young adulthood, one has acquired, as it were, a tentative level of the sense of coherence, a picture of the way the world is. One now makes major commitments: marriage and a new nuclear family; the work at which one will spend most of one's waking hours; a style of life; a set of social relationships. These provide one with a relatively stable set of life experiences, day after day and year after year. By the time a decade or so has passed, if not sooner, the tentativeness has been transformed into a considerable degree of permanence. One selects and interprets experiences to conform to the established level of the sense of coherence. It is unlikely, then, that one's sense of coherence, once formed and set, will change in any radical way. Fluctuations will be minor.

But unlikelihood is not certainty, which brings us to the second part of our answer to the question about the dynamic nature of the sense of coherence: modification of the sense of coherence. We can point to two major ways in which an adult's sense of coherence can undergo fairly significant transformations. First, there is the cataclysmic stressor, in either a broad or a personal sphere, which transforms a great variety of life experiences, often in a brief period of time, through a considerable change in one's GRRs (Arrow B). One has had no hand, no choice, in this experience and often no preparation for it. Perhaps the classic example is sudden widowerhood. War, forced migration, the death of one's child, losing one's job because the plant closed down, a natural disaster—central to all these events is not primarily that they are largely unanticipated, in a personal sense, but that they bring in their wake a variety of unpredictable experiences. Inevitably, then, they result in a significant weakening of one's sense of coherence.

Is such weakening necessarily permanent? To ask this question is to point to the second major way one's sense of coherence can undergo a significant modification. By contrast to the first, it is never sudden, almost always has an element of choice (conscious or unconscious), and can result in movement in either direction on the sense-of-coherence continuum. Let us take widowerhood as an example. Whatever one's previous level of sense of coherence, this is inevitably a major disruption of one's life, particularly when there has been no anticipatory socialization. Slowly and painfully, one can choose experiences that, offering meaningful stimuli, rebuild one's sense of coherence. Or, if one is lucky, such experiences are thrust on one. No less can the opposite pattern characterize one's life (see Parkes, 1972; Parkes, Benjamin, and Fitzgerald, 1969). In parallel fashion, and not necessarily as a result of a cataclysmic stressor, a woman can go out to paid work after decades of being a housewife; an illiterate person can learn to read and write; one can undergo psychotherapy; one can embark on a substantially different kind of work; one can marry or divorce. Change, then, can take place. But change of this type is always within the context of one's previous level of the sense of coherence, is always slow, and is always part of a web of life experiences that transmit stimuli that are more or less coherent. Movement toward the strong end of the continuum always requires hard work.

Generalized Resistance Resources

If one's life experiences, then, shape one's sense of coherence, what shapes one's life experiences? What determines whether they consist of coherent or incoherent stimuli and are characterized by consistency, participation in shaping outcome, and neither underload nor overload? Part of the answer—the effect of stressors—was given above (Arrow B). But the greatest part of my answer is one's generalized resistance resources (Line C). GRRs are discussed in great detail in Chapter Four. By definition, a GRR provides one with sets of meaningful, coherent life experiences. Thus Line C is a symbol more for tautology than for causality. If material resources or a flexible coping strategy or social supports by definition provide coherent life experiences, if that is their hallmark, one cannot quite say that the relationship is causal, for there is no way of testing the truth of the statement. The value, however, of separating GRRs from life experiences in the diagram, and the meaning of Line C, is that we are thereby provided with a theoretical criterion, a culling rule, for identifying GRRs. The empirical prediction, which can be tested, is the relationship between GRRs and the sense of coherence, which can be defined and measured independently.

At the present stage in the development of the salutogenic model and without considerable empirical research, we have no basis for predicting the structure of the relationship between GRRs and the sense of coherence. Is a given GRR—for example, a clear, stable ego identity or social supports—a necessary or even a necessary and sufficient condition for a strong sense of coherence? Or, if such generalizations are impossible, are some GRRs more useful than others in coping with certain stressors (Arrow D, Figure 1)? One of the advantages of the salutogenic model is that it allows us—indeed, even stimulates us—to ask such questions, whatever the answers turn out to be.

Sources of GRRs

We can now move further "back" in the diagram. Arrows E point to the sources of the GRRs. These have been discussed at length in Chapter Five. I would only briefly point up a number of issues that may have been slighted earlier. First, whatever the somewhat cavalier approach I may seem to have taken with regard to the role of stressors in influencing health status, I did so only to offset the strong current concern with stressors. As will be evident shortly, this position must be qualified. I take it here in order to point out that there are also direct links between the sources of GRRs and stressors (Arrow F). Someone growing up and living in a society with an annual per capita income of $250 confronts different stressors and has different GRRs at his or her disposal than does someone growing up and living in a society with a per capita income of $2,500. Living in a world with limited means of transportation and communication and weapons of destruction is quite different from living in a "civilized" world of satellites, 747s, and nuclear weapons. Whether one's society has pacific or hostile relations with its neighbors matters a great deal both for the GRRs and the stressors in one's life. It is perhaps even more important, in these terms, to distinguish between people who are members of different social classes, sexes, or ethnic groups within one society.

Second, I see no grounds for assigning priority to one or the other of the two major sources of GRRs (childrearing patterns and social-role complexes) in shaping the GRRs at one's disposal. At first sight, it might seem clear that there is a greater affinity between childrearing patterns and ego identity and between present social class position and material resources. But ego identity and adult major role activity and role set are deeply intertwined, as are parental social class and present material resources. The relationships, then, are complex. Then again, they may well be not as complex as seems to be the case. There is at least some reason and empirical evidence to think that there is a wholeness in the direction in which one is constrained to go by the complex of one's childrearing patterns and social-role complexes, in a given sociocultural and historical setting. The strain toward consistency among these acts to push one in the direction of a greater or lesser degree of GRRs. This consistency enables us to speak of the prototypical life chances of an individual in a given subculture—for example, of a poor, white housewife in Appalachia.

The relationship between cultural and individual factors brings us to a third point. Whatever the very major power of sociocultural and historical factors in shaping the GRRs at one's disposal, we are witness to substantial individual differences. Intelligence, however it may be measured, is distributed on a normal curve. Beauty, charm, strength, and a myriad of other personal characteristics, however these are measured, vary from person to person. Of course these are measured and evaluated differently in different cultural settings. Of course they are influenced and perceived differently depending on the social context. But these idiosyncratic characteristics and tendencies are not therefore irrelevant in shaping the GRRs at one's disposal. One can make reasonable probabilistic predictions knowing a person's sociocultural world as to where he or she will rank on GRRs. But the prediction will never be close to perfect for a given individual.

Finally, we must note the role of chance as a source of GRRs. The luck that confronts us is often far from a matter of luck. Further, one person may take advantage of a lucky opportunity while another may not. One may even be so strong a determinist as to claim that everything that happens had to happen. There are,

nonetheless, chance events that may often be of considerable significance in shaping one's GRRs. Rarely does one buy a sweepstakes
ticket, chat with a stranger while waiting for a train, register for a
class because it is held at a convenient hour, leaf through the personal ads in a magazine, or get invited to a party and thereby embark on a chain of events that substantially alters one's life. Rare.
Far less important than childrearing patterns and social-role complexes. But it does happen.

Stressors

Let us now assume that we have accounted adequately for
the emergence of a given level of the sense of coherence that characterizes a person at a given time and return to the center of the
diagram. Before we can explicate the relationship between the sense
of coherence and health, we must focus on the place of stressors in
the salutogenic model. I touched on this issue above in considering
the impact stressors can have on GRRs (Arrow B). Now we look
elsewhere.

Chapter Three opened with a statement pointing to the evidence of the relationship between stressors and movement toward
the dis-ease end of the health ease/dis-ease continuum. This statement requires some clarification. Biochemical and physical stressors—
droughts, bombings, invasion, pests—much as psychosocial stressors,
can have an impact on GRRs. But unlike psychosocial stressors,
whose impact is always mediated through GRRs and the sense of
coherence, biochemical and physical stressors can be of such direct
traumatic magnitude as to bypass interaction with the sense of coherence. A noxious gas, a poisonous substance, a bullet, or a car can
act directly on the health status of an individual (Arrow G; double
arrow shows two-way causation). Alternatively, a cumulative harsh
overload of such stressors (smoking or exposure to asbestos or to
high noise levels) can act indirectly on health by exploiting the
endogenic potential pathogens and "weak links" in interaction with
a state of stress (Arrow H; double arrow shows interaction).

There is, indeed, good reason for the pathogenic model to
have dominated thinking about disease for most of human history.
The three-pronged power of stressors (Arrows B, G, and H), which

included perhaps above all nutritional deprivation and the most primitive level of sanitation, was sufficient to overcome even substantial resistance resources.[1] When, however, the standard of living in a society (or in some segments of a society) reaches a rough level of adequacy, differences in health level no longer are overwhelmingly determined by biochemical and physical stressors. At this point psychosocial stressors and, above all, the sense of coherence become crucial variables. And at this point salutogenesis becomes at least as intriguing and important a question as pathogenesis.

Management of Tension

Having analyzed the sense of coherence as a dependent variable, we now turn to consider it as an independent variable. The achievement of a roughly adequate standard of living does not do away with physical and biochemical stressors. They remain ubiquitous. For the first time in history on a large scale, however, it has now become possible to cope with them. Success has been remarkable. The triumphs of public health and of the microbiological sciences have been great (Arrow I). But there is a built-in limitation, which Dubos (1960) has profoundly analyzed. The bugs, as I have put it, are smarter. Not always, not every bug, and they have retreated. In this era of chronic diseases (and not much less applicable to infectious diseases in such an era) the single-bullet approach can no longer be seen as viable in and of itself or even as the dominant weapon. In this context the sense of coherence becomes important.

As shown in the model, the role of the sense of coherence is three-directional. First, by mobilizing the GRRs at one's disposal (Arrow D), as well as specific resistance resources (SRRs), a strong sense of coherence can avoid one's being subjected to some stressors (Line J). Second, it allows us to define some stimuli, which others might perceive as stressors, as innocuous or even as welcome (Line K). But whether we like it or not, none of us can in such ways keep

[1] Yet even during the worst plagues, some remained healthy and some recovered. Had our focus been salutogenic, we might have learned much more about GRRs than we know today. For a brilliant if tongue-in-cheek paper analyzing the remarkable plague immunity of an ethnic minority in ancient Egypt thanks to a powerful GRR technically called Bohbymycetin, see Caroline and Schwartz (1975) on chicken soup.

stressors out of our lives. Day in, day out, throughout our lives, we find that stressors put us repeatedly in a state of tension (Arrow L). Periods of calm and stability, of homeostasis, are rare in human existence. At this point the third direction in which a strong sense of coherence operates is decisive. It would hardly be important were stressors reducible to an occasional experience (which is almost never the case), much as it is not very important when stressors are overwhelming. We respond to a state of tension, if we have a strong sense of coherence, by mobilizing those GRRs that we have at our disposal and that we judge to be appropriate in seeking to resolve the tension by overcoming the stressor (Arrow M; double arrow shows interaction). (See Pearlin and Schooler's 1978, pp. 6–7, discussion of the three functions of coping responses: to modify situations, to control the meaning of situations, and to control the stress.)

We can now clarify the dual function of GRRs. Earlier we noted their function in creating life experiences that produce a strong sense of coherence. In this sense, they are constantly active. But they also function as a potential. Someone with a strong sense of coherence, whatever its sources, confronted with tension, can call on the GRRs to manage the tension successfully. One brings to bear one's wealth, one's knowledge, one's strong ego identity, one's social supports, and so forth. Note that this approach does not obviate the need for GRRs of the internal environment to perform a holding action. Physical and biochemical resources are required to prevent too rapid a transformation of tension into stress (Selye's stage of exhaustion). But the crucial role of GRRs is in overcoming the stressor and thereby resolving the tension. One must add that the person with a strong sense of coherence can also directly mobilize SRRs appropriate to the particular stressor. Finally, it bears repeating in the present context that overcoming a stressor and resolving tension is a life experience that in turn reinforces the sense of coherence (Arrow N). By overcoming a stressor we learn that existence is neither shattering nor meaningless.

From a dynamic, historical point of view, the dual function of GRRs can now be seen as one. Since conflict and stressors are ubiquitous throughout life and hence tension is at least as characteristic of human beings as is homeostasis, one is from earliest infancy calling on whatever GRRs are at one's disposal. When they suffice to provide a life experience that makes sense to us—that is consistent with our expectations, allows us some participation in determining outcome, and has neither too few nor too many stimuli for us to handle—and thus allow us to resolve tension, another building block is added to our sense of coherence. This theoretical approach, it should be noted, underlies my analysis of the relations between people and communities and the health care institution in Chapter Eight.

Stress

Given the initial statement of the problem as that of salutogenesis, there remains but one issue to consider at this point, the feedback impact of health status. That is, in the never-to-exist society in which people are never harmed by traumatic or cumulative physical and biochemical insults, protected as they are by public and private health measures; in which all persons have a very strong sense of coherence and hence are capable of mobilizing GRRs and SRRs—in such a never-never land, one knows much tension but never stress. And so all would be on the extreme ease end of the health ease/dis-ease continuum, at least until one emulates Oliver Wendell Holmes' wonderful one-horse shay in a dramatic ending. Over and over again, we would manage tension successfully, thereby reinvigorating our sense of coherence (Arrow N) and at least maintaining our easeful health status (Arrow O). But given the brilliance of the bugs and the inevitable inadequacies of the sense of coherence and of exogenous GRRs, even the most fortunate are bound, on occasion, to fail to manage tension well. Cousins, it will be recalled, did come down with ankylosing spondylitis. Freud did suffer from cancer of the jaw.

There is no need here—particularly since I do not intend to deal with theories of diseases—to discuss the relationship between a state of stress and movement toward the dis-ease end of the health continuum (Arrow P). This is the focus of attention of almost the entire stress literature. I can make no contribution. Of far greater significance, the thrust of this entire book is to propose a shift in concern to the study of successful tension management. Two points are germane here.

First, it seems clear to me that stress is a general precursor.

Only when stress interacts with the existing potential endogenic and exogenic pathogens do pathological consequences occur (Arrow Q). As Selye puts it (1975, p. 41) (notwithstanding his unclear use of the word *tension*): "Although stress itself is defined as the 'non-specific response of the body to any demand,' the weakest link in a chain will be the one that selectively breaks under tension. Similarly, the weakest part of any animate or even inanimate machine will be the one that fails when a nonspecific, general demand is made upon the performance of the whole." A most important corollary of this approach is the rejection of the concept of psychosomatic disease. Other than the massive traumata that leave none unscathed (Arrow G), all diseases are usefully understood as psychosomatic. In other words, almost all breakdown involves stress. Stress, however, does not determine the particular expression of the breakdown.

My second point is crucial to the salutogenic approach. The pathogenic orientation asks: What causes a person to become ill with a particular disease? The salutogenic orientation, by contrast, asks: Whatever the person's particular location at any given time on the health ease/dis-ease continuum, what are the factors that facilitate his or her remaining at that level or moving toward the more salutary end of the continuum? Thus no assumption is made that one is well and becomes sick. On the contrary, the commitment is to seeing people at some point on the health continuum at any given time and continually confronted with stressors and hence with the problem of preventing tension from becoming stress. In this way, the sense of coherence is always hypothesized to be a relevant factor.

Health

Which brings us to the final issue. Heretofore, we have viewed one's location on the health ease/dis-ease continuum as a dependent variable. We have seen it as the final outcome of a long chain of phenomena. Such analytic albeit complex neatness is distorting. One's health status can be usefully viewed as an independent variable in three ways. First, it can affect the extent to which one is exposed to stressors (hence Arrow G points in both directions). At a high health level, conflicts in social relations may be attenuated or phase-specific crises borne with equanimity. Second, good health is in itself a significant generalized resistance resource by the definition of a GRR as a factor that fosters meaningful and sensible life experiences. Third, in the same way that the other GRRs are interrelated, being on the healthy end of the health continuum can facilitate the acquisition of other GRRs (Arrow R).

Throughout, and particularly in the final section of Chapter Two, I have insisted that the health ease/dis-ease continuum is not to be regarded as coextensive with the entire realm of well-being. Other ease/dis-ease continua exist. To have entered into a systematic discussion of what these continua are, how our locations on them are determined, and how they relate to our concern with health would have been an impossible and unnecessary task within the scope of this book. Suffice it to say, then, that a nod has been made in their direction; they are highly relevant to and intertwined with health, but they are distinct. If our interest is in understanding health, then location on the family-relations or social-relations or material-resources ease/dis-ease continua can usefully be viewed as a GRR.

Reality, for better or for worse, is complex. The attempt to understand reality of necessity oversimplifies in that it must select and abstract. In this chapter, I have sought to minimize such oversimplification. Hence the perhaps bewildering array of arrows and lines and boxes in Figure 1. Doubtless the attempt has fallen short in one sense or another. Thus, for example, I have certainly dealt inadequately with genetic and constitutional GRRs and with public and private health measures. Genetic and constitutional GRRs are too complex and are beyond my capacities to explore here; public and private health measures are considered in Chapter Eight and in the Epilogue. I would be troubled, however, only if the central paradigm of the book was not clear. This paradigm finds its graphic expression in the diagram. Stripped of all qualifications and complexities, the thick lines in the diagram and the italicized words in its key are what I have to say.

Chapter Eight

Implications
for an Improved
Health Care System

Let me make my position clear at the outset of this chapter, which discusses the implications of the salutogenic model for relationships of individuals and groups with health workers and the health care system. I do not in this chapter pretend to have any instant therapy or guide to the perplexed. In my discussion of the sense of coherence I have viewed it as a deeply rooted, pervasive orientation. I have located its sources primarily in childrearing patterns and social-role complexes and have described it as developing and being reinforced over the course of many years. To blame a weak sense of coherence, as many do, on doctors or the health care system is sheer demonology. A culture tends to manifest a strain toward consistency. If, indeed, many of the pressures impinging on a given population group are in the direction of forming a weak sense of coherence, then it is likely that its members' experiences with health care workers and the health care institution will point in the same direction. It is easy but fruitless to play the game of blaming the doctors. The precise opposite is no less true. To imagine that the individual health worker or health care institutions in general can go far in fostering a strong sense of coherence when other social institutions pressure in the opposite direction is illusory.[1]

The Patient and the Health Care System

Having said this, however, is not at all tantamount to saying that the nature of the life experiences of persons acting within the health care system has no relationship to the sense of coherence. This relationship can be analyzed on three levels: traumatic situations; incremental and relatively slight reinforcement or weakening of the sense of coherence; and the more significant impact of the health care system in the community. But before these are analyzed, a number of preliminary considerations are in order.

First, we are concerned with the prototypical patterns of encounters and not with the idiosyncratic relationship that may develop between a patient and a doctor. That relationship is shaped largely by personality factors. Personality factors do, of course, enter any particular relationship, whether barefoot doctors or Harley Street consultants, confused adolescents or strong longshoremen are involved. But the arena for play of personality, by and large, is not that great. Close observation of large series of encounters or relationships would reveal systematic patterns that are shaped by struc-

---

[1] In this paragraph, I have referred interchangeably to doctors and to other health care workers. It will be awkward to continue to do so. I will, therefore, refer only to doctors. In principle, my analysis of the relationship between the individual (or family) and the doctor can include relationships with nurses, dentists, medical social workers, and so forth or with health care teams. In practice, for good sociological reasons, the physician is most often central in the relationship even when authority is delegated to others. Another terminological difficulty is the use of the word *patient*. Given the fact that our health care system is predominantly a disease care system, the word *patient* implies that the person is in some way sick. In the framework of the health ease/dis-ease continuum, what I mean by patient is anyone who is in a reciprocal role relationship with a physician, whatever the location on the continuum. Below I use particular terms for patients and for doctors as indicative of the particular type of role relationship.

tural and cultural factors. Hence our central question is not the moral, What should be the relationship? nor is it the abstract, What can it be? Rather, we shall ask, Given a certain normative relationship between person and health worker, what are its consequences?

Second, if consequences, then one must specify consequences for what. We are not concerned with an overall analysis of the functions of the patient-doctor relationship. The dependent variable in this chapter is the sense of coherence. The case has been argued that a person's sense of coherence is a major variable in the determination of his or her health status. Let us assume that this has been demonstrated. To the extent, then, that what the doctor does or does not do influences a patient's sense of coherence, it thereby affects his or her state of health.

Third, and of most importance, my analysis is best understood in the context of the theoretical model of salutogenesis. As a teacher of medical students, I have often put it that I view my role as training one type of generalized resistance resource, the doctor. But I can now see, in retrospect, that though it sounded good—the doctor would help his patients fight all the ubiquitous bugs with the particular weapons at his disposal—it was a fuzzy notion. I did not understand why resistance resources are important and how they deal with stressors. Once one adopts the concept of the sense of coherence, the link becomes clear. The doctor, as a potential GRR, has the possibility of structuring life experiences for people that reinforce their sense of coherence. If encounters with the health care system indeed systematically are characterized by consistency, participation in shaping outcome, and an underload-overload balance of stimuli, the sense of coherence is maintained or reinforced.

But note that the word *potential* has been used. As I pointed out in Chapter Four, some GRRs, stood on their heads, can weaken the sense of coherence. This is true for doctors. There is no need to exaggerate. A patient with a strong sense of coherence will not emerge from encounters with doctors, whatever their nature, with a significant change. But this is not to say that there can be no impact. The matter, rather, is one for empirical study. What must be remembered is that inherent in all such encounters, to a greater or lesser extent, are anxiety, uncertainty, unpredictability, and dependence.

Traumatic Situations. I have tried to place the assessment of the potential impact of the patient-doctor encounter on the sense of coherence in proper proportions. Consideration of the anxiety and dependence inherent in the encounter, however, brings us to situations in which the nature of the encounter can have a fairly decisive influence on the sense of coherence. Such situations may constitute a small fraction of the over one billion (in the United States) encounters that take place annually between patients and doctors. But absolutely they do involve a substantial number of people and are the most dramatic and memorable encounters.

Let us take two examples. The first almost invariably involves interaction with the physician; the second may or may not. In Chapter Seven, I noted that one's location on the health ease/dis-ease continuum may have a feedback impact on one's GRRs. A woman who has undergone a mastectomy, someone who has had a leg amputated or has suffered a stroke or severe burns often confronts the danger of rapid radical erosion of the sense of coherence. True, one's pretraumatic level is a decisive variable in determining what will happen. Some people may have so strong a sense of coherence that even such a trauma has a blunted impact. But, for many, the word *shattered* is appropriate. The physician, I suggest, can in such situations—since he or she is in any case closely involved—play a significant role in the slow, painful, and difficult task of reestablishing the sense of coherence.

The second example is a bit more complex and bears a direct relationship to the nature of the health care system. Traumatic psychosocial stressors can have a direct impact on GRRs (Arrow B in Figure 1). I have already alluded to the studies showing the sharply increased mortality rates of widowers in the six months following death of the wife. Whatever the strength of one's sense of coherence, a fairly sudden, radical change in one's GRRs—ranging from a chemical engineer aged fifty-two losing his job to a loyal member of the Communist Party confronted with Khrushchev's speech at the Twentieth Party Congress—has the potential of rocking the foundations of a sense of coherence. A personal or structured relationship between doctor and patient or a health care system that institutionalizes channels for providing information of such traumata to personnel opens the possibility for the contribution of the physician in reestablishing the sense of coherence.

The literature on what has come to be called crisis intervention is vast. Much thinking (though precious few randomized control trials) has been invested in how the health and other well-being services can contribute to the welfare of people in such situations. What has been lacking, I believe, is a theoretical understanding of what happens to people who go through such situations. Conceptualizing the process as the disintegration and reintegration of the sense of coherence via concern with the life experiences provided by GRRs, I submit, may open the way for possible intervention. (For an important analysis of the possible role of the physician in such situations—an analysis that is most congruent with the concept of the sense of coherence—see Parkes, 1972.) The conditions under which reintegration is more or less likely to occur are best analyzed by looking at the routine encounter.

Routine Encounters. It bears repeating to say that, whatever the individual variation from patient to patient and situation to situation, predominant modes characterize the interaction of any one doctor with his patients and indeed of patient-doctor interactions in any given sociocultural setting. Three elements present in all settings influence this regularity.

First, the patient invariably perceives the situation as involving anxiety, uncertainty, and ambiguity. In our terms, the life situation of patient-doctor interaction is inherently antithetical to a sense of coherence. This perception may vary in intensity from that experienced during a routine checkup to that experienced in an interaction with perceived critical consequences for health outcome. But even in the most innocuous situation, few patients show total equanimity.

Second, the fact that a person has entered the interaction means that he or she has acknowledged that the doctor has a particular technical competence in dealing with certain kinds of problems— a competence that the patient does not have. Even in situations where entry is involuntary (compulsory examinations in industry, the military, prison), one finds such acknowledgement, though the doctor may be perceived in different terms from the way a doctor is perceived in a voluntary situation. The doctor always assumes a relatively superior professional competence.

Third, there is an inevitable built-in difference in the perspectives of the patient and of the doctor. The patient always normatively is concerned with his or her self-interest, whatever the cultural limits of propriety may be in a given setting. The doctor can never, Parsons notwithstanding, be solely concerned, normatively, with the patient's self-interest. (Parsons' stress on the collectivity orientation was first formulated in Parsons, 1951, chap. 10. In his latest comments on the subject, in 1978, there is no indication that he has revised his position.) This is not a matter of a possibly different perception of the patient's self-interest. The extent to which other concerns impinge on the doctor's orientation can vary greatly. But even in the most extreme situation—the physician, privately employed by a monarch or tycoon, who has thoroughly internalized the norm of "for the good of the patient"—the doctor must keep one eye out for his or her own welfare. Other than in these rare situations, the doctor always has commitments to other patients, to his or her other roles, to norms relating to not being taken in or exploited. Such norms are based on the unwritten obligation the physician has assumed toward society, in return for some degree of professional autonomy, to minimize the social costs of illness. This obligation is most often taken to mean to cure the patient; but it also involves a stance against malingering and the like (see Merton, 1976, p. 68).

Though Illich has not explicitly analyzed the doctor-patient relationship in these terms, it would be consistent with his position to argue that handing over responsibility for coping with anxiety to the doctor, acknowledging the doctor's technical competence, and the doctor's being concerned with interests other than those of the patient are key factors in iatrogenesis. "The main source of pain, of disability, and of death is now engineered, albeit nonintentional, harassment. Our prevailing ailments, *helplessness* and injustice, are largely the side effects of strategies for more and better education, better housing, a better diet, and better health" (Illich, 1976, p. 262; my emphasis). But his blanket, prophetlike indictment obscures rather than enlightens the analysis of the structural modalities of the doctor-patient relationship that influence the sense of coherence of the patient.

Given the above three elements in the relationship, which modalities foster restoration or maintenance of the sense of coherence and which weaken it? We now turn to this question.

Perhaps the most eloquent confrontation with the problem of anxiety is Eric Cassell's 1976 book. He distinguishes between illness and disease. Illness refers to what the patient feels is wrong; disease refers to what medicine says is wrong. The physician's responsibility, Cassell argues, is to deal with both problems, to heal and to cure. The thrust of Cassell's argument is that it is much more humane and decent for the physician to accept this dual burden rather than limit himself or herself to the responsibility for curing. Among the core elements of illness he describes are a loss of the feelings of omnipotence, of connectedness, and of personal indestructibility and also a loss of the power of rational reasoning and of the sense of control (pp. 30–44). The relationship between these elements and the sense of coherence is self-evident. If indeed the sense of coherence is related to curing, then it follows that, for the physician to cure, he or she must cope with the problem of a lessened sense of coherence. Cassell does not make this connection explicitly. His argument rests essentially on moral rather than on theoretical, instrumental grounds.

But his very humaneness makes him oblivious to a substantial danger. Cassell's choice of extreme vocabulary—omnipotence, personal indestructibility—is misleading. He seems to suggest that these feelings characterize us when we are well and that the physician's responsibility is to restore us to such a grand state. The physician is obviously much closer, both because he is well and because he is a physician, to such a state. This belief can lead, though unintentionally, only to urging the patient to see the physician as omnipotent and to place faith and fate in his or her hands. And indeed, Cassell is at his most comfortable and most humanely moving in his writing on the terminal patient, for whom there is no hope at all of returning to omnipotence, connectedness, and the other extreme characteristics.

Cassell's analysis, then, is double edged. The physician-patient relationship is structured, as he would have it, by the doctor's concern for the total patient as a person, total commitment to all the needs of the patient, and assumption of ultimate responsibility for meeting these needs as best as is humanly possible. There is little doubt that such a relationship is at least consonant with the characteristics of life experiences that I have argued foster a strong sense of coherence. Cassell would be extremely sensitive to assuring that the interaction with the patient is consistent and contains an appropriate load balance (of information, for example). He is explicitly careful to assign maximum participation to the patient in doing things for himself or herself, much as God requires a great deal of the believer.

There are, however, three pitfalls in this approach that inevitably prevent the reestablishment of the sense of coherence. First, while God or the parent of the small child may be omnipresent, the doctor is not, even for the terminal patient. The patient, socialized into decision-making dependence, is helpless when the physician is not present. From the point of view of the sense of coherence, there are undoubtedly situations in which this mode of relationship is completely appropriate. Szasz and Hollender (1956) refer to the activity-passivity model in clinical situations of anesthesia, acute trauma, coma, delirium, and so forth. The only possible road to a return of the patient's sense of coherence in such situations is physician decision making. But most physician-patient interactions, particularly in an era when both prevention and chronic illness are increasingly important, are not of this type. In such cases, a relationship that leaves decision making in the hands of the physician can only impair the sense of coherence.

The second pitfall refers to ignoring the cultural context of the relationship. We are dealing with a situation of faith in the omnipotence of the physician as the basis of restoration of the sense of coherence. Such faith is inherent in therapy administered by God or by His sacred representatives. It is quite efficacious in a cultural context where God is omnipresent or when the patient is, for some temporary period, in a total patient role being cared for by sacred representatives, as well as in the clinical situations referred to above. But when the patient is expected to be an adult in his or her other role relationships, when the culture puts a premium on decision making by oneself, such a structured role relationship with the physician is dysfunctional because it violates the need of patients, in certain cultural contexts such as those of Western societies, to equate participation in determining outcome with decisional and not only behavioral participation.

The issue, moreover, goes even further than participation in decision making. Patients arrive at the encounter, having been shaken by their illness, with an attempt at restoring their sense of coherence. They do so, implicitly or explicitly, by casting their illness in a subjectively sensible etiological, diagnostic, prognostic, and therapeutic framework. When doctor and patient share a common language, as is the case in much non-Western medicine, the patient can find only confirmation. But often, in situations where doctors and patients are from different social class and cultural backgrounds, the medical belief systems of the two differ. The doctor most often does not even inquire into the patient's belief system. When the doctor fails to do so and acts solely within the system of scientific medicine, which is often not even congruent with the patient's system, the awesome omniscience of the physician can only confuse the patient.

Engel (1977) has put Cassell's case for healing in a far more sophisticated and ethically neutral way. The tendency to reduce medical action to the biomedical sphere not only disregards the psychic needs of the patient, which are, in the patient's view, legitimate medical problems, but makes it impossible to adequately understand even supposedly straight somatic problems. Only when the doctor sees and relates to the patient as a person in a sociocultural context can the results of interaction be effective from the point of view of the patient as well as of the doctor.

The approach of Cassell and Engel, then, in rejecting a narrow, somatic, biomedical conceptualization of the appropriate scope of the patient-doctor encounter, fosters the sense of coherence. Engel does not fall into the trap of positing the omnipotent doctor, inimical to the sense of coherence in a Western cultural context. But he, like Cassell, also ignores a third pitfall that follows from broadening the scope of the interaction. They both disregard the problem of power in the relationship. The patient not only is anxious but, by definition, is dependent. By entering into the relationship, the patient has acknowledged the legitimacy of the dependence, though perhaps with ambivalence. Broadening the scope of the interaction to include the doctor's viewing the patient as a total person increases the dependence. The power relationship, then, is inherently asymmetrical. By ignoring this issue, Cassell and Engel are saying: Place your trust in the doctor (and in the professional group that monitors its members' behavior) that he or she will not exploit the asymmetry.

At this point, it is appropriate to recall the third inherent element in the doctor-patient relationship. The doctor can at the most only temporarily suspend his or her other commitments and devote himself or herself to the needs of the patient. In other words, there are always the temptation and the pressure to take advantage of the asymmetry. This can be done in many ways. At one extreme, the patient can be exploited financially or for the ego gratification of the doctor or sexually. In academic centers, the patient can be used for teaching and research purposes not in the immediate interest of the patient. At the gentlest extreme, the doctor can act in consideration of other patients.

I am not saying that such advantage is always taken. Nor am I raising a moral issue. I am saying that the inherent nature of the relationship not only makes taking advantage possible but pressures in this direction. What is important in the present context is that the extent to which the doctor's behavior is perceived by the patient as anything other than in the total interest of the patient is bound to weaken the sense of coherence. The crucial test is not that of diagnosis or therapy proposal but rather that of decision making. The patient who has the opportunity of saying "Go ahead" or "Stop" or of saying "I trust you enough to accept your proposal" or "You haven't yet gained my trust" is in a life experience characterized by participation in determining outcome.

Let me put my point in another way. Patients are always instrumentally dependent on the doctor, for they need the doctor to give them what they believe they cannot, for whatever reason, get for themselves. The possibility of power dependence is thereby created, for patients can never fully judge what is being done for their own good. But the doctor can never act solely for a patient's good. Unless counteracted, the consequences for the patient's sense of coherence are detrimental. (For a most helpful set of theoretical analyses based on data and germane to this section, see Ben-Sira, 1972, 1976.)

Modalities. We have, in part implicitly, in part explicitly, considered the question of how the life experience of the patient-doctor encounter can be characterized by a high or low degree of consistency, participation in shaping outcome, and an underload-overload balance. Three crucial factors have been identified as shaping this life experience: scope of legitimate expertise, ranging from a narrow, specific focus on the technical, somatic presenting problem to perception of the patient as a total person in a sociocultural context; goals of interaction (assuming that the patient always focuses on his or her needs), ranging from the doctor's nearly total focus on needs of other than the patient to total focus on the patient's needs as perceived by the patient; power allocation, ranging from total decision-making power in the doctor's hands to total decision-making power in the patient's hands.

The consequences for the sense of coherence are not simple. The more the patient is perceived as a total person, the better. The more the focus is on the needs of the patient, the better. The more decision-making power rests in the hands of the patient, the better. However, in the real world fundamental structural properties of the doctor-patient relationship—built-in characteristics of the relationship independent of the particular patient and particular doctor—militate against such possibilities.

It becomes, then, helpful to depart from the general concept of the doctor-patient relationship and to confront different possible modalities or types of relationships. Having clarified the issues involved, we can now ask: Which modality offers the best opportunity for the most efficacious interaction to take place from the point of view of the sense of coherence? Parsons (1978) proposes a set of four models of social organization. His argument that the collegial modality is the most appropriate way of conceptualizing the doctor-patient relationship need not concern us here. I will spell out the details of the models, as I understand them, in the terms of the above discussion. The labels used are mine, in the hope that they clarify. I have also added what seems to me to be a crucial fifth type. The details appear in Table 7. It is, I trust, clear that categorization is only for the sake of simplicity in presentation. No concrete interaction is ever a pure type but only tends in one direction or the other.

A concrete doctor and a concrete patient can establish a relationship that is not governed by the pressures of this or that modality, thereby obtaining the advantages of this one and avoiding

Table 7. Alternative Conceptualizations of the
Doctor-Patient Relationship

Type	Parties	Scope of Legitimate Expertise	Patient's Need Satisfaction Is Primary[a]	Decision-Making Power
Market	Consumer-purveyor	Specific technical presenting problem	No	Shared
Bureaucratic	Client-professional	Specific technical presenting problem	No	Not in patient's hands
Democratic, friendship	Partner-partner	Unlimited	Yes	Shared
Collegial	Patient-practitioner	Specific technical presenting problem	Yes and no	Not in patient's hands
Sacred	Layperson-divine (priest)	Unlimited	Yes	Not at all in patient's hands

[a] In all cultures, the patient, whatever the modality, legitimately assigns primacy to his or her own need satisfaction. Thus the modalities differ only in the aims of the interaction in the doctor's eyes.

the dangers of that one. By and large, however, consistent patterns tend to be laid down that are well described by this set of alternatives. What, then, are the implications of each modality for the patient's sense of coherence?

The relationship that conforms to the *market* modality tends to be quite destructive. It is governed by the doctrine of caveat emptor. It is functional for the patient's sense of coherence in that the patient—in the theoretical pure-market situation—can legitimately shop around, ask questions, and insist on sharing decision-making power, always being able to turn to an alternative purveyor of health care services. In this sense, the current trend in some quarters, particularly in the United States, to speak of the patient as a consumer is salutary. But the price to be paid is highly dysfunctional. The doctor is pressed to care for his own interests, only qualified partially by the norm of "in the interest of the patient." The consumer can rarely have a consumers' rights organization sufficiently present in the concrete situation to allay the anxiety and is pressed to mistrust the doctor. Further, the doctor inevitably focuses on his or her area of technical expertise; it takes too much uncompensated time and energy to consider the total person.

The *bureaucratic* modality is, if anything, more detrimental to the sense of coherence of the patient. This negative effect has nothing to do with the pejorative implications of the term. Trained incapacities, Parkinson's Law, red tape, and the like in a bureaucratic context only exacerbate the dysfunctional consequences inherent in the doctor-patient relationship. The very nature of the context compels the physician to adhere to norms and rules established in the interest of patienthood but not necessarily of the individual patient or of the organization. The amorphous idea of the patient as a whole person is anathema to the classification required by bureaucratic organization. The client's rights and duties are spelled out but by the organization. The only possible countervailing force to such pressures is the establishment of institutionalized procedures and structures explicitly designed to limit and direct the power of the organization—for example, when a trade union owns or sets up a health care service for its members. This solution, however, creates its own problems, such as the "proletarianization" of the physician (McKinlay, 1978). The iron law of oligarchy should make us skeptical of whether such a countervailing force can solve the problem of decision-making power.

The *democratic,* or *friendship,* modality, visualizing a physician-patient partnership, on the face of it seems most likely to promote a sense of coherence. In this modality, the physician must be altruistic, subordinating all other interests to the patient's needs. The relationship, being personal, is by definition all embracing and not limited to the technical problem. Power is shared and decisions are made jointly, with all the cards on the table. But, to continue the metaphor, there are two crucial jokers. First, so personal a relationship inevitably militates against the affective neutrality that is essential if the physician is to meet the central technical requirements. The physician, in diagnosis and formulation of proposals for therapy, cannot do well if he or she is too emotionally bound up with the patient. The issue is even more clearly seen when one considers the inevitable reality of patients toward whom the physician has negative emotions—bias, dislike, disrespect. To ask the physician to be affectively neutral only with regard to his negative emotions is a contradiction in terms. Second, the democratic modality disregards an essential property of all doctor-patient relationships. Though the degree may vary, the patient is always dependent. To ask full partnership in exercising decision-making power is to place an intolerable overload on the patient. Even a physician, when he or she enters the patient role, is subjectively incapable of assuming the burden of decision making. Anxiety inevitably prevails over technical knowledge. And, unlike the case in the market modality, the patient cannot easily terminate the relationship.

Parsons proposes that the *collegial* modality "is the most appropriate and the most likely to have a strong prospect of survival in the field of purveying of professional services" (1978, p. 452). He does not say appropriate for what. We may infer that he means that this modality is the most adequate conceptualization of the reality of the practice of American medicine. This may well be true. It may even be the modality most likely to survive in the United States. But it is not necessarily the most conducive to a strong sense of coherence.

Cassell's analysis, considered above, is one of the most forceful expressions of the collegial relationship at its most humane. He has transcended, as noted, two of the limitations that I believe are inherent in the collegial modality, namely, a focus on the specific technical problem and only partially according primacy to the patient's need satisfaction. Such transcendence is evidently possible but only because of unusual individual characteristics and motivations. The collegial relationship by its nature promotes dealing with the technical problem, for, after all, this is the particular realm of special expertise that is the basis of the claim of physicians for professional autonomy and that brings the patient to the physician in the first place. That collegial physicians have been trained in teaching hospitals with a strong technical orientation may be a historical accident. I return to this issue later. But even Cassell has not transcended a third limitation, namely, that decision-making power in the collegial modality remains in the physician's hands. This is in the terms of the contract. The doctor is the expert and knows what is best for the patient. In a sense, the collegial physician who transcends the other limitations, thereby gaining the full trust of the patient, paradoxically impinges on the possibility of sharing decision making with the patient. One does not share power with God. Damage is inevitably inflicted on the patient's sense of participation in determining outcome. But this analysis of the situation must be qualified; in subcultures or cultures fully accepting God or His representatives as the physician, such damage is not inevitable.

Which brings us to the final modality, the *sacred* relationship. Limited to thinking in American middle-class terms, Parsons does not realize that the layperson-divine mode (divine in the sense of priest rather than godlike) not only must be included in a systematic typology of modalities but is empirically found in all parts of the world, including the fortress of Western scientific medicine. The tremendous advantage for the sense of coherence of this modality derives from the complete cultural congruence between patient and doctor. Whether Christian Scientists, Taiwanese, Ethiopians, or from Sri Lanka, the patient and doctor fully share conceptualization of etiology, classification of illness and disease, probable course, appropriate therapy, and so on. The doctor still remains the expert but is a medium who has been blessed. (See Kleinman, Eisenberg, and Good, 1978; Obeyesekere, 1973; and Young, 1976b, 1977.)

The sacred relationship, then, would seem to be the modality that most powerfully fosters restoration of the patient's sense of coherence. The patient's anxiety and emotional needs are fully taken care of, and he or she is related to as a total person. The patient, appropriately socialized, has complete faith in the doctor's commitment to the primacy of his or her needs. Though decision-making power is not in the patient's hands, this is not at all troubling. Carefully prescribed behavior, following doctor's orders, assures the sense of participation in determining outcome.

The sacred mode, when practiced in a cultural context to which it is appropriate—where there is total faith in God or the gods and in representatives of divine power—does not present the dangers noted in the discussion of Cassell's work. But Cassell works with an armamentarium that is far more efficacious in coping with somatic diseases than are all other forms of medical practice, the romantic debunkers of what we know as scientific medicine notwithstanding. In other words, in the world of reality, those who practice the sacred mode, no matter how much they are concerned with healing, are not all that good at curing. Does this not damage the sense of coherence? Not at all, for what must be understood is that patients at home in such a modality have a ready-made and totally self-convincing explanation for such failure. Often, the patient's faith has been inadequate. Young points to a more profound understanding when he notes that our mistake is that we attempt "to study all medical beliefs as attempts to control events within the bodies of sick persons instead of studying them in the contexts of phenomenological reality and the division of labor in society" (1976a, p. 147).

The failure to cure, then, is not the Achilles' heel of the sacred modality from the point of view of the sense of coherence. It would be, in my view, the most powerful modality in restoring the sense of coherence for those with complete faith were it not for the inherent danger of abuse. When all decision-making power is in the hands of the divine, the sense of coherence is not impaired as long as the layperson maintains complete faith. But divines are people. They have inevitable tendencies to perceive themselves as the Divine. This is compounded by two further tendencies. First, the inherent uncertainty of medical practice, in the face of the need to act, gives rise to anxiety. Second, absolute power raises the possibility of corruption—of abandoning the primacy of the patient's interests. Unless these tendencies are controlled, the chances are considerable that the patient will perceive the fallibility of the doctor (see Freidson, 1970). When this happens, the negative consequences for the sense of coherence are substantial.

We have now considered five modalities of the doctor-patient relationship. There are, as we have seen, considerable advantages to all but the bureaucratic mode for the sense of coherence of the patient. (This mode, though, has advantages from other points of view.) One might, then, think that the individual physician, alert to the importance of the problem of the patient's sense of coherence, would structure a modality that selects the best of all possibilities and avoids its pitfalls. Within narrow limits, this is indeed possible. But the limits are narrow. The physician, after all, works within a health care system and a broader social structure that impose considerable constraint. It is to this system and structure that we now turn.

Impact of the Health Care System and the Social Structure

It would be manifestly impossible here to attempt an intricate analysis of how the health care system in any given society shapes the dominant modalities of the physician-patient relationship. (An important but not very integrated endeavor in this direction is found in Gallagher, 1978, and particularly in McKinlay's paper therein.) I shall, therefore, only raise a number of issues that seem to me to be most pertinent to the subject of this book.

A good starting point is the dominant system of medical education. Of the 900-odd medical schools in the world, almost all have adopted the ideal of living in the post-Flexnerian world. This is not that much less true of the training institutions for other health care workers. I do not in the least denigrate the significance and achievements of scientific medicine. But two inherent characteristics of training in an academic, scientific institution have major implications for the modality of the doctor-patient relationship. First, the enormous achievements of biomedical science are most consonant with a focus on the specific technical, somatic presenting problem of the patient and make adoption of the democratic or sacred modalities difficult. Engel (1977), who has put the case against the narrow biomedical orientation with so much sophistication, has not asked himself why this model is adhered to with so much tenacity.

Second, training for scientific medicine is closely integrated with teaching hospitals and academic research institutions. Clinical experience, then, is centered overwhelmingly on the horizontal patient, most often with a complex somatic disease. Not only do such patients constitute an unrepresentative sample of the patients in the overwhelming number of doctor-patient encounters; but they are by definition in a bureaucratic setting. The patient is learning material. On all three counts—scope of legitimate expertise, primacy of patient's need satisfaction, and decision-making power—the student is best prepared for the bureaucratic modality.

Moving out into the real world, the young physician faces one of three dominant alternatives, depending on the society in which he or she lives. In a world increasingly committed to societal provision of health care to its citizens as a right, the physician more and more becomes a salaried employee of a bureaucratic organization, a niche for which training has been most appropriate. Alternatively, in capitalist societies, the market model is culturally most appropriate. But the contractual terms imposed, exchanging professional autonomy for normative commitment to the best interests of the patient, often make the physician uncomfortable in the market modality. The rewards of being the supreme culture hero—all studies of occupational prestige assign pride of place to the physician—are contingent on behavior conforming to this norm. There is, then, pressure to adopt the collegial modality and play God. This is even more true in those societies, such as those of most of Western Europe, where the market modality is attenuated by sick funds (private, public, or governmental) and contractual arrangements with individual physicians or an organized group of physicians.

The cultural world of the Western physician is a secular world. It has its magic, its rituals, and its superstitions, but the sacred is reserved for special days and special buildings, which do not include the hospital or doctor's office. Hard science reigns supreme, as an ideal. In such a world, the sacred modality has little place. It is identified with "quackery"—Christian Science, homeopathy, faith healers, snake-oil salesmen, and the like. This is not to say that practitioners of the sacred modality do not exist. Quite the contrary is true. This very fact pressures the "legitimate" physician to stress the scientific character of the medical profession all the more. Whatever the temptation to become a divine, the physician must set himself off from the "quacks." Inevitably this requirement leads one to steer clear of such murky notions as the whole person and to focus on the soma, with which one is most comfortable.

In these and other ways, then, the particular social structure—capitalist, welfare capitalist, social democratic, authoritarian communist—and the particular value system in which the physician has been educated and within which he or she works shape the structural properties of the doctor-patient relationship. This is, of course, only one side of the coin. The patient too contributes to the shaping of the relationship. Here matters are far more complex, for patients from different social classes, with different ethnic backgrounds and social roles, have different expectations and value orientations. Thus, for example, the physician with a largely upper-middle- or upper-class patient population is likely to share decision-making power with the patient. He or she often assumes that the patient's capacity for information load is large. Lower-class patients are likely to elicit an assumption on the part of the physician that because they have different vocabularies, facility in language, capacity for abstraction, and the like, they are incapable of participation in determining outcome.

We now turn briefly to what may well be, in the long run, the most significant consequence of the practice of medicine (and of other health care professions) for the sense of coherence. Our entire discussion so far has focused on the doctor-patient encounter. Given the fact that the average person in the industrialized world has some four or five such encounters each year, the impact cannot be dismissed, though it should not be exaggerated. But such encounters of doctor and patient are overwhelmingly limited, in most countries of the Western world, to what is so erroneously called the health care system. The more appropriate term is the disease care system, as I have noted in Chapter Two. The encounter is almost by definition between a patient and a doctor oriented to treating a disease and to disregarding dis-ease, not to talk of ease.

I have now come full circle to the salutogenic orientation. Overwhelmingly, the medical profession is organized, intellectually and structurally, to assume responsibility for curing a disease when the patient enters the disease care system. It would be futile, unwise, and inhumane to argue that this should be otherwise. Those who do enter this system are the people who hurt most, who are most in danger of dying. The thrust of my argument, however, has been that a salutogenic orientation and the sense of coherence are not luxurious frills. To ignore them is to be self-defeating. Perhaps health care is not simply a matter of frantically plugging holes in dikes. I deal with this long-range issue in the Epilogue. But a care system that is organized to deal only with breakdown is a system that can no longer make serious advances.

I shall leave to others, or to myself elsewhere, the question of what form of broader social organization is most conducive to a strong sense of coherence, even though this question is the most overriding one. Nor do I think it appropriate to urge doctors qua doctors to become involved in revolution, social work, social engineering, and so forth. But at both the group and individual level and given the assumption that the sense of coherence is related to health, one must ask: Can the medical profession and the individual physician engage in activities beyond the patient-doctor encounter that affect the sense of coherence? I would suggest four major activities that can positively affect the sense of coherence: making health care available to all, promoting a preventive health orientation, buttressing trust in the physician, and reaching out to persons at high risk of damage to the sense of coherence.

I would start with what seems to me to be the underlying value premise at the broadest possible level. In my original "breakdown" paper, even before I had formulated the concept of the sense of coherence, I wrote (Antonovsky, 1972, p. 542): "The ties between an individual and his total community are decisive resistance resources. One indicator of such ties would be the extent to which a society holds as a central value that the society as such, rather than the individual alone, is responsible for dealing with threat or for assisting the individual to do so." A society, then, that has institutionalized a health care system that expresses consensus that health care is an inalienable right of all its citizens and is to be made equally available to all on the universalistic ground of being a resident of that society is a society that has taken a step forward in strengthening the sense of coherence of its members. If one is blocked from access to health care because one is poor or a member of a racial minority or lives in a rural area, one's image of the world as coherent—given the importance of health in people's lives—is necessarily impaired.

Second, it will have been noted that one of the generalized resistance resources included in Figure 1 is a preventive health orientation. Doctors are not the only source of this orientation, but surely the profession as such can play a key role in facilitating its adoption. Again, what is important is not so much the action of individual physicians as the institutionalized mechanisms for health education, highlighting of risk factors, facilities for early detection, and so forth. It seems reasonable to posit that strengthening of this GRR contributes to a strong sense of coherence.

The third issue to be raised at the supraindividual level refers to the image of the physician in society. This issue has been dealt with, in a broader context than just that of the medical profession, in *The Limits of Benevolence,* by W. Gaylin and others. In a review of the book, we read (Starr, 1978, p. 9): "Progressive reformers assumed a coincidence of values and interests between caretakers and the dependent and were willing consequently to entrust professionals with enormous discretionary authority. Today, reformers increasingly assume a potential conflict between benevolent institutions and their clients." The more the medical profession is trusted, in the simplest of terms, the more likely is a population to have a strong sense of coherence. The role of the mass media is not to be discounted; both heroic exploits of doctors in saving lives on television programs and headlining malpractice suits have their effects. But far more important, in my judgment, are such matters as the perception of unwarranted income levels, costs of health care, opposition to or promotion of health-insurance programs, concern with environmental hazards, readiness for self-policing, and availability for public scrutiny. The medical profession is always likely to be a bearer of trust, whatever the barbs of Molière and George Bernard Shaw, more than any other occupational group. There is, however, a considerable margin. The level of trust, at any given time in history, can affect the sense of coherence.

The fourth and final issue, like the issue of a preventive health orientation, derives from the salutogenic framework. I refer to the availability of institutionalized mechanisms to identify high-risk groups but in a broader than usual sense. A high-risk group is generally thought to consist of those who smoke, are poorly nourished, are old, are exposed to noxious agents, and the like. In the present context, my concern is with those people subject to particular stressors that have adversely affected their generalized resistance resources. Thus, the widower, the adult who loses a job, the parents of a child who has died may not break down directly, but their sense of coherence is affected. Note that I have not here suggested that the medical profession as such can deal with poverty, unemployment, racial discrimination, migration, or other socio-historical sources of a weak sense of coherence. My point, rather, refers to the structured lines of communication between the doctor and the population for which he or she is responsible. With a structured mechanism for acquiring such information, the doctor can reach out at a time when more good might well be done than when the consequences of the trauma become manifest.

There is no need to discuss the role of the individual physician in making health care available to all in the community, in promoting a preventive health orientation, in buttressing an image of trust in the physician, and in reaching out to high-risk persons. Whether he or she works in this direction in some measure depends on the individual personality and value system. But it depends far more, as does the direction of action or inaction of the medical profession, on the society in which the profession operates and on the social structure of health care delivery and its ideological premises.

I explicitly stated at the outset of this chapter that I had no intentions of writing a guide to the perplexed. I have discussed a number of issues that seem to me to be central in relating the sense of coherence of people to the policies and practices of medicine (and, by implication, of other health professions). I have discussed these issues in what is essentially a sociological frame of reference, which is at least one appropriate way of understanding what doctors do and can do in strengthening the sense of coherence of patients and potential patients—that is, of all of us. I have avoided dealing with many complex issues of health and health care not directly related to the central themes of the book. Above all, I have raised questions and not insisted on answers. If those who more directly than I bear the responsibility for health care take up the challenge and begin to formulate answers, such was my intention.

Epilogue: Outlook for Human Health

The central problems with which this book is concerned—survival and the quality of life in the realm of health—have been with us for a long time. Survival was the central health concern throughout most of human history and in much of the world it remains central even today. But the direction for successful coping with this problem is reasonably clear, as difficult as it may be to move in this direction for socioeconomic reasons. In the industrialized world, however, we are approaching the limits of life expectancy in large populations. As Burnet puts it (1971, pp. 154, 168; see also all of his chap. 8), "The 'allotted span' for any species is something genetically programmed as a result of evolutionary processes. . . . Nature is not going to cooperate with us in keeping men or any other animal alive for much beyond the span she has allotted."

If this is indeed the case, then neither the sense of coherence nor any other factor is of much relevance for the survival of those who are near the allotted span of years, at least on an overall population basis. At first sight, it would seem that the real health problem in industrialized societies is that of "premature" death. Not that any death is seen as "mature," at least in our culture. But when early deaths in one group—blacks, poor people—are more frequent than in another group, there is good reason to apply the concept of premature deaths. With the advent of chronic diseases as the major cause of early mortality, the real health problem of industrialized societies becomes the quality of life.

The issue, then, I would discuss in this concluding chapter is that of the implications for the future of the analysis presented in this book. It is, I think, useful to put this discussion in the context of the presentation of the four most outstanding thoughtful considerations of the question that have emerged in recent years. In doing so, I follow the lead of Thomas McKeown's Rock Carling Fellowship monograph (1976, pp. 160–180). After summarizing the major approaches of Lewis Thomas, René Dubos, and Ivan Illich, and that of McKeown himself, I will discuss the expectations for coming decades that flow from the salutogenic model.

Thomas (1974, pp. 36–42), representing most contemporary biomedical scientists, distinguishes among three levels of technology in medicine. When diseases are not understood, all medicine can do is provide the supportive therapy that tides patients over, presumably until they recover or die. As indispensable as the therapy is from a human point of view, its cost is extremely high. Once this investment was largely in the infectious diseases; now the chronic diseases require it. But it is no more than a holding operation, used because medicine does not know what else to do. The second level of technology is the hospital-based, enormously expensive, "highly sophisticated, and profoundly primitive" technology of transplants, coronary-care units, chemotherapy, and the like. This technology is designed to make up for the ravages of disease or to postpone death. Again, at the human level, Thomas cannot reject such expenditures.

Neither of these activities, in Thomas' view, is of significant utility in promoting advances in the health level of the population. Real hope is to be placed in the third level of technology in medicine, which is based on a genuine understanding of disease mechanisms. We now can deal effectively with diphtheria and bacterial infections, syphilis and tuberculosis, and various nutritional disorders because we have gained this understanding. This effective technology also has the virtue of being quite cheap. For Thomas, the application of basic knowledge has been the basis of major advances in health levels in the past and is the direction that is quite promising for the future. "If I were a policy maker," he concludes (p. 41), "interested in saving money for health care over the long haul, I would regard it as an act of high prudence to give high priority to a lot more basic research in biologic science."

Dubos, no less a distinguished biological scientist than Thomas, only in part shares his analysis of the past and his prognosis for the future. It is true, he writes (1968, pp. 100–101), that "many of the most destructive diseases of his [Benjamin Franklin's] time have now been brought under control. The application of these methods [of modern medical science] to disease control offers such diversified potentialities that one can anticipate scientific solutions for almost any medical problem, once it has been clearly defined." There are, however, three central reasons, in Dubos' view, for being critical of Thomas' position. First, the position rests on the doctrine of specific etiology or, as Dubos has put it, the mirage of the magic bullet (1960, pp. 91ff.). The etiology of chronic diseases is complex and can be understood only in terms of multiple causation. Whatever the utility of Thomas' approach in the past, it is not likely to be of much help in the future. Second, Dubos stresses the fact that "economic, social, and ethical difficulties often complicate or prevent altogether the practical utilization of existent knowledge for the prevention and treatment of disease" (1968, p. 101). But perhaps the most important thrust of Dubos' position is his third observation, that "each period and each type of civilization will continue to have its burden of diseases created by the unavoidable failure of biological and social adaptation to counter new environmental threats" (quoted in McKeown, 1976, p. 163).

Dubos prefers to see himself as a "moderate optimist" (1973, p. 184). Clearly, he rejects Thomas' faith in the future, which rests on the advances of biological science. But his own faith is equally strong. Humanity will surely, he argues, find the will to work out the conscious social and economic arrangements required to replace the previous "spontaneous adaptive processes" in meeting new challenges. Dubos relies on the "ground swell of dissatisfaction" expressed by businessmen and scientists and in the countercultures of youth, as well as on the historical precedents of the rise of Islam and Christianity, which he sees as examples of humanity's capacity to adapt to new challenges (1973, chap. 12).

While Thomas explains the advances of the past and bases his hopes for the future in the realm of the biological sciences, and Dubos, although with a tempered appreciation of the past contribution of scientific medicine, places his faith in humanity's adaptive capacities, Illich lays the crucial disease problems of contemporary industrial society at the doors of the disease care institution. Illich is a priest by calling and very much of a catholic (small *c*) scholar. He first sounded his thesis in a general discussion of technological development in modern society (1973). In looking at the past, he grants that for a brief period from about 1913 through World War II, modern medicine had some effective treatment to offer, as did many shamans and herb doctors; and this treatment made a modest contribution to man's well-being. But, by the mid 1950s, it became clear that it is "the malignant expansion of institutional health care [that] is at the root of the rising costs and demands and the decline in well-being. . . . Society can have no quantitative standards by which to add up the negative value of illusion, social control, prolonged suffering, loneliness, genetic deterioration, and frustration produced by medical treatment" (1973, pp. 6–7).

Illich's devastating, well-documented, and detailed attack on medicine (1976) quickly became a best seller. As McKeown summarizes Illich's position (1976, pp. 166ff.), modern medicine is thrice iatrogenic in that "medicine does more harm than good; it breeds demands for its services and supports features of society which generate ill health; most seriously, it diminishes the capacity of the individual to deal with his own health problems and to face suffering and death."

Illich can be understood only as a prophet. It is his mission to denounce the sins of Sodom and Gomorrah, not to qualify and measure. As for the past, he is not concerned with a balanced appraisal and assignment of credit but only with showing how the technological institutionalization of medicine and of modern life bears negative consequences for our health. Others will praise achievement; the prophet's mission is to strip bare our illusions and sins.

For Illich, then, the medical establishment, with the brain-washing it has wrought in modern society, is the Devil. We must learn not only to be stoical in the face of the inevitable pain and misery of life but also to see how they are rewarding. Thus implicit in Illich's position is the view that even if we manage to free our-selves from social and cultural iatrogenesis, our health status is not likely to improve. The only real strand of hope in his outlook is found in his attack on medical iatrogenesis. In the unlikely event that the Western scientific medical institution is abolished, people will at least not be subjected to the damage done to our health by turning to doctors.

McKeown's own position contrasts sharply with the views of the men he discusses. His view of medicine (1976) is not as dream (Thomas), mirage (Dubos), or nemesis (Illich). In the distant past, the major dangers to health were those determined by the primitive conditions of life: food shortage, homicide, accidents, and predation. Then, with the agricultural revolution some ten thousand years ago, infectious diseases joined inadequate nutrition as the predominant cause of sickness and death. With the significant improvement in the last century in the standard of living and particularly in nutritional standards, as well as in public health control of the environment, major strides in health status have been made.

Today we face a somewhat different set of problems, but McKeown believes that his analysis of the past points the way to the conditions that must be met to allow us to cope with new problems. As he puts it (1976, p. 100; compare p. 174): "Those fortunate enough to be born free of significant congenital disease or disability will remain well if three basic needs are met: they must be adequately fed; they must be protected from a wide range of hazards in the environment; and they must not depart radically from the pattern of personal behavior under which man evolved, for example by smoking, overeating, or sedentary living."

If we are, then, to avoid premature death and improve the health quality of our lives, we must follow the two major paths of the past century: reasonable nutritional standards and control of environmental hazards. But the relatively new great challenges of the chronic diseases are best met in the realm of personal behavior. Thus, for example, he writes, "In the past century the improvement in expectation of life of mature males from all causes has been reduced by at least half by smoking alone" (p. 99). Thus McKeown does not see as the key to the future Thomas' commitment to biological sciences, Dubos' faith in man's social adaptive capacities, or Illich's hostility toward the medical establishment. His stress is on concrete changes in behavior on the individual level, and he would have us change our eating, smoking, and exercise habits. "As these are now the main determinants of health, it is hard to believe that society will not wish to create conditions under which such practices are encouraged" (p. 164).

I do not deny the importance of the views presented above. Basic biological research will provide us with immunological and therapeutic weapons against specific diseases. Dubos' stress on multiple causation and the need to study the conditions under which endemic microorganisms become pathogenic and his orientation to the social determinants of the application of scientific knowledge, vague as it is, are important contributions to our thinking about disease. Illich's concern with undermining the legitimacy of concentration of power in the hands of the disease care establishment opens the way for a useful skepticism. And certainly McKeown's rational, data-guided approach is in the best empirical tradition of attacking concrete dangers.

But much as all four positions share the fundamental virtue of going beyond the narrow emphasis on what doctors do today as the key to hopes for improvement of the health quality of life, they all are characterized by fundamental inadequacies. Thomas' position is most open to criticism, which has been effectively leveled by Dubos. The notion of the conquest of disease after disease by magic bullets is doubly illusory: first, because chronic diseases can be understood only in terms of multiple causation; second, because the bugs are smarter. Illich has no real answer, except that we should learn to live with our suffering. At best, he urges us to stay away from doctors, thus at least avoiding iatrogenic diseases. Mc-Keown disregards not only the difficulties of changing behavior but also the data that show that the behaviors he would change account for only a small part of the variance in disease causation.

The basic inadequacy of Thomas and McKeown, however, is conceptual. Theirs is a pathogenic orientation. Their central question is that of the etiology of diseases, in Thomas' case, or of disease as well as diseases, in McKeown's. Hence they inevitably focus on the elimination of disease agents. Illich, curiously enough, shares this medical bias. He differs only in identifying the major disease agent as the medical establishment.

Dubos, however, opens the way for a radical reconsideration of the problem. Not only does he, with Illich, assume that the bugs will always be with us. Not only does he draw our attention to the social-cultural-economic context in which the bugs flourish and become virulent. But he also raises the question of our capacities for adaptation and the social determinants of these capacities. This is the heart of what I have called the salutogenic orientation. Dubos' profound insights, his humanity, and his moving fluency, however, do not lead him to go beyond posing the question. Clearly, my own thinking has been strongly influenced by Dubos' work; I have tried to go beyond what he has done.

The sense of coherence, I have argued, is a central component of the answer. The stronger the sense of coherence of individuals and groups, the more adequately will they cope with the stressors immanent in life, and the more likely are they to maintain or improve their positions on the health ease/dis-ease continuum. In Chapter Eight, I dealt with the possible impact of the doctor-patient relationship and of the dominant modes of disease care delivery on the sense of coherence. But, as noted there, this realm is hardly the decisive arena of life experience.

The real issue is whether the societies in which our children grow up and in which we live our daily lives facilitate or impede the development and maintenance of a strong sense of coherence. Do they provide us with the generalized resistance resources that give us experiences of an appropriate underload-overload balance of stimuli, of consistency, and of participation in the shaping of outcome? For most of us, I would suggest, such life experiences—at our paid work, in our housework, in our social relations, in relation to our community—are not at all frequent.

Of course it matters very much where one is located in the social structure. Social classes, ethnic and racial groups, men and women do not all share the same set of life experiences. To generalize about national societies without awareness of the great difference it makes whether one is an Appalachian coal miner, a suburban upper-middle-class housewife, or a university professor is to obscure any possible understanding of differences in the sense of coherence.

If we wish to see the present and future soberly in our world, we must use words like *capitalism* and *totalitarianism*. The social structures in which most of humanity lives and the daily experiences to which we are exposed in these structures are far from conducive to a strong sense of coherence. This observation is as true for the United States as for the Soviet Union, for China as for India. Societies with a marketing mentality and a fetishism of commodities, with terror and arbitrary recasting of history, with grinding poverty and starvation cannot foster a view of the world as one that provides information and music except for the fortunate few.

It would take another book and an extensive research effort to subject to serious analysis the concrete social structures and social positions that in our world foster a strong sense of coherence. Improvement in health status is contingent on such analysis and on a program of social action that could follow. The analysis is one of the crucial tasks of social epidemiological research. The task, however, cannot be undertaken unless there is an adequate set of conceptual tools at our disposal. To provide such a set of tools has been the central purpose of this book.

References

ALEXANDER, F. *Psychosomatic Medicine: Its Principles and Applications.* New York: Norton, 1950.

ANDREWS, F. M., AND WITHEY, S. B. "Developing Measures of Perceived Life Quality: Results from Several National Surveys." *Social Indicators Research,* 1974, *1,* 1–126.

ANDREWS, F. M., AND WITHEY, S. B. *Social Indicators of Well-Being: Americans' Perception of Life Quality.* New York: Plenum, 1976.

ANTONOVSKY, A. "The Ideologies of American Jews: A Study in Definitions of a Marginal Situation." Unpublished doctoral dissertation, Department of Sociology, Yale University, 1955.

ANTONOVSKY, A. "Toward a Refinement of the 'Marginal Man' Concept." *Social Forces,* 1956, *35,* 57–62.

ANTONOVSKY, A. (Ed.). *The Early Jewish Labor Movement in the United States.* New York: YIVO Institute for Jewish Research, 1961.

ANTONOVSKY, A. "Social Class and Illness: A Reconsideration." *Sociological Inquiry,* 1967a, *37,* 311–322.

ANTONOVSKY, A. "Social Class, Life Expectancy and Overall Mortality." *Milbank Memorial Fund Quarterly,* 1967b, *45,* 31–73.

ANTONOVSKY, A. "Social Class and the Major Cardiovascular Diseases." *Journal of Chronic Diseases,* 1968, *21,* 65–106.

ANTONOVSKY, A. "Social and Cultural Factors in Coronary Disease: An Israel–North America Sibling Study." *Israel Journal of Medical Sciences,* 1971, *7,* 1578–1583.

ANTONOVSKY, A. "Breakdown: A Needed Fourth Step in the Conceptual Armamentarium of Modern Medicine." *Social Science and Medicine,* 1972, *6,* 537–544.

ANTONOVSKY, A. "The Utility of the Breakdown Concept." *Social Science and Medicine,* 1973, *7,* 605–612.

ANTONOVSKY, A. "Conceptual and Methodological Problems in the Study of Resistance Resources and Stressful Life Events." In B. Dohrenwend and B. Dohrenwend (Eds.), *Stressful Life Events: Their Nature and Effects.* New York: Wiley, 1974.

ANTONOVSKY, A. (Ed.). *Abraham David Katz: Jew, Man, and Sociologist.* Jerusalem: Israel Institute of Applied Social Research, 1975.

ANTONOVSKY, A. "Letter to the Editor." *American Scientist,* 1978, *66,* 272–274.

ANTONOVSKY, A., AND ARIAN, A. *Hopes and Fears of Israelis: Consensus in a New Society.* Jerusalem: Jerusalem Academic Press, 1972.

ANTONOVSKY, A., AND BERNSTEIN, J. "Social Class and Infant Mortality." *Social Science and Medicine,* 1977, *11,* 453–470.

ANTONOVSKY, A., AND HARTMAN, H. "Delay in the Detection of Cancer." *Health Education Monographs,* 1974, *2,* 98–128.

ANTONOVSKY, A., AND KATS, R. "The Life Crisis History as a Tool in Epidemiologic Research." *Journal of Health and Social Behavior,* 1967, *8,* 15–20.

ANTONOVSKY, A., AND KATS, R. "The Model Dental Patient: An Empirical Study of Preventive Health Behavior." *Social Science and Medicine,* 1970, *4,* 367–380.

ANTONOVSKY, A., AND LORWIN, L. (Eds.). *Discrimination and Low Incomes.* New York: New York State Commission Against Discrimination, 1959.

ANTONOVSKY, A., AND SHOHAM, I. *Social Resistance Resources and Health in Middle Age.* Jerusalem: Israel Institute of Applied Social Research, 1978.

ANTONOVSKY, A., AND OTHERS. "Epidemiologic Study of Multiple Sclerosis in Israel. I: An Overall Review of Methods and Findings." *Archives of Neurology,* 1965, *13,* 183–193.

ANTONOVSKY, A., AND OTHERS. "Twenty-Five Years Later: A Limited Study of the Sequelae of the Concentration Camp Experience." *Social Psychiatry,* 1971, *6,* 186–193.

ANTONOVSKY, H., AND ANTONOVSKY, A. "Commitment in an Israeli Kibbutz." *Human Relations,* 1974, *27,* 303–319.

BAHNSON, C. B. "Role of the Ego Defenses: Denial and Repression in the Etiology of Malignant Neoplasm." *Annals of the New York Academy of Sciences,* 1966, *125,* 827–845.

BAHNSON, C. B. "Epistemological Perspective of Physical Disease from the Psychodynamic Point of View." *American Journal of Public Health,* 1974, *64,* 1034–1040.

BECKER, E. "Review of Tiger and Fox' *The Imperial Animal." Transaction/SOCIETY,* 1972, *9,* 40–43.

BECKER, H. *Outsiders: Studies in the Sociology of Deviance.* New York: Free Press, 1963.

BELLOC, N. B., BRESLOW, L., AND HOCHSTIM, J. R. "Measurement of Physical Health in a General Population Survey." *American Journal of Epidemiology,* 1971, *93,* 328–336.

BEN-SIRA, Z. "The Doctor-Patient Relationship: Collectivism or Exchange?" Unpublished doctoral dissertation, Department of Sociology, Hebrew University, 1972.

BEN-SIRA, Z. "The Function of the Professional's Affective Behavior in Client Satisfaction: A Revised Approach to Social Interaction Theory." *Journal of Health and Social Behavior,* 1976, *17,* 3–11.

BENSMAN, J., AND ROSENBERG, B. *Mass, Class, and Bureaucracy.* Englewood Cliffs, N.J.: Prentice-Hall, 1963.

BERKMAN, L. F. "Social Networks, Host Resistance and Mortality: A Follow-Up Study of Alameda County Residents." Unpublished doctoral dissertation, Department of Epidemiology, School of Public Health, University of California, Berkeley, 1977.

BERKMAN, L. F. "Psychosocial Factors, Host Resistance and Mortality." *American Journal of Epidemiology,* in press.

BLUM, H. L., AND KERANEN, G. M. *Control of Chronic Diseases in*

Man. Washington, D.C.: American Public Health Association, 1966.

BOOTH, A., AND COWELL, J. "Crowding and Health." *Journal of Health and Social Behavior,* 1976, *17,* 204–220.

BOWLBY, J. "The Making and Breaking of Affectional Bonds." *British Journal of Psychiatry,* 1977, *130,* 201–210, 421–431.

BRESLOW, L. "A Quantitative Approach to the World Health Organization Definition of Health: Physical, Mental, and Social Well-Being." *International Journal of Epidemiology,* 1972, *1,* 347–355.

BRIDGES-WEBB, C. "The Traralgon Health and Illness Survey." *International Journal of Epidemiology,* 1973, *2,* 63–71; 1974, *3,* 37–46, 233–246.

BRINTON, C. *The Anatomy of Revolution.* Englewood Cliffs, N.J.: Prentice-Hall, 1965.

BRONFENBRENNER, U. (Ed.). *Influences on Human Development.* Hinsdale, Ill.: Dryden, 1972.

BUCKLEY, W. (Ed.). *Modern Systems Research for the Behavioral Scientist.* Chicago: Aldine, 1968.

BURNET, M. *Natural History of Infectious Disease.* Cambridge, Great Britain: Cambridge University Press, 1953.

BURNET, M. *Genes, Dreams, and Realities.* Aylesbury, Bucks, Great Britain: Medical and Technical Publishing Co., 1971. (Also New York: Basic Books, 1971.)

BURNET, M. *Intrinsic Mutagenesis: A Genetic Approach to Aging.* New York: Wiley, 1974.

CANNON, W. B. *Bodily Changes in Pain, Hunger, Fear, and Rage.* New York: Appleton-Century-Crofts, 1929.

CANNON, W. B. *The Wisdom of the Body.* New York: Norton, 1939. (Revised and expanded edition, 1963.)

CAPLOVITZ, D. *The Poor Pay More.* New York: Free Press, 1963.

CAROLINE, N. L., AND SCHWARTZ, H. "Chicken Soup Rebound and Relapse of Pneumonia." *Chest,* 1975, *67,* 215–216.

"Case Records of the Massachusetts General Hospital." *New England Journal of Medicine,* 1977, *297,* 828–834.

CASSEL, J. "Psychosocial Processes and 'Stress': Theoretical Formulation." *International Journal of Health Services,* 1974, *4,* 471–482.

CASSEL, J. "The Contribution of the Social Environment to Host Resistance." *American Journal of Epidemiology,* 1976, *104,* 107–123.

CASSEL, J. "The Relation of the Urban Environment to Health: Toward a Conceptual Frame and a Research Strategy." In L. E. Hinkle, Jr., and W. C. Loring (Eds.), *The Effect of the Man-Made Environment on Health and Behavior.* Atlanta: Center for Disease Control, Public Health Service, 1977.

CASSEL, J., PATRICK, R., AND JENKINS, D. "Epidemiological Analysis of the Health Implications of Culture Change: A Conceptual Model." *Annals of the New York Academy of Sciences,* 1960, *84,* 938–949.

CASSEL, J., AND TYROLER, H. A. "Epidemiological Studies of Culture Change. I: Health Status and Recency of Industrialization." *Archives of Environmental Health,* 1961, *3,* 25–33.

CASSELL, E. J. *The Healer's Art: A New Approach to the Doctor-Patient Relationship.* Philadelphia: Lippincott, 1976.

Center for Disease Control. *Reported Morbidity and Mortality in the United States: Annual Summary 1977.* DHEW Publication No. CDC78-8241. Atlanta: Public Health Service, 1978.

CHAN, K. B. "Individual Differences in Reactions to Stress and Their Personality and Situational Determinants." *Social Science and Medicine,* 1977, *11,* 89–103.

COBB, S. "Social Support as a Moderator of Life Stress." *Psychosomatic Medicine,* 1976, *37,* 300–314.

COBB, S., AND ROSE, R. M. "Hypertension, Peptic Ulcer, and Diabetes in Air Traffic Controllers." *Journal of the American Medical Association,* 1973, *224,* 489–492.

COCHRANE, A. L. *Effectiveness and Efficiency: Random Reflections on Health Services.* London: Nuffield Provincial Hospitals Trust, 1972a.

COCHRANE, A. L. "The History of the Measurement of Ill Health." *International Journal of Epidemiology,* 1972b, *1,* 89–92.

COLLEN, M. F. *A Case Study of Multiphasic Health Testing.* Oakland, Calif.: Permanente Medical Group and Kaiser Foundation Research Institute, 1977.

Commission on Chronic Illness. *Chronic Illness in a Large City:*

The Baltimore Study. Cambridge, Mass.: Harvard University Press, 1957.

COSER, L. *The Functions of Social Conflict.* New York: Free Press, 1956.

COSER, R. L. "The Complexity of Roles as a Seedbed of Individual Autonomy." In L. A. Coser (Ed.), *The Idea of Social Structure: Papers in Honor of Robert K. Merton.* New York: Harcourt Brace Jovanovich, 1975.

COUSINS, N. "Anatomy of an Illness (as Perceived by the Patient)." *New England Journal of Medicine,* 1976, *295,* 1458–1463.

CROSSMAN, R. (Ed.). *The God That Failed.* New York: Harper & Row, 1950.

CUTLER, S. J., AND YOUNG, J. L. "Demographic Patterns of Cancer Incidence in the United States." In J. F. Fraumeni (Ed.), *Persons at High Risk of Cancer.* New York: Academic Press, 1975.

DAHRENDORF, R. *Class and Class Consciousness in Industrial Society.* Stanford, Calif.: Stanford University Press, 1966.

DATAN, N. "Women's Attitudes Toward the Climacterium in Five Israeli Sub-Cultures." Unpublished doctoral dissertation, Committee on Human Development, University of Chicago, 1971.

DATAN, N., ANTONOVSKY, A., AND MAOZ, B. *A Time to Reap: The Middle Age of Women in Five Israeli Subcultures.* Baltimore: Johns Hopkins University Press, forthcoming.

DATAN, N., AND GINSBERG, L. H. (Eds.). *Normative Life Crises.* New York: Academic Press, 1975.

DOBZHANSKY, T. *Evolution, Genetics, and Man.* New York: Wiley, 1955.

DODGE, D. L., AND MARTIN, W. T. *Social Stress and Chronic Illness: Mortality Patterns in Industrial Society.* Notre Dame, Ind.: University of Notre Dame Press, 1970.

DOHRENWEND, B., AND DOHRENWEND, B. (Eds.). *Stressful Life Events: Their Nature and Effects.* New York: Wiley, 1974.

DORN, H. F., AND CUTLER, S. J. *Morbidity from Cancer in the United States.* Monograph No. 56. Washington, D.C.: Public Health Service, 1959.

DUBOS, R. J. *The Mirage of Health.* London: Allen & Unwin, 1960.

DUBOS, R. J. "The Evolution of Microbial Diseases." In R. J.

Dubos and J. G. Hirsch (Eds.), *Bacterial and Mycotic Infections of Man.* (4th ed.) Philadelphia: Lippincott, 1965.

DUBOS, R. J. *Man, Medicine, and Environment.* New York: Praeger, 1968.

DUBOS, R. J. *A God Within.* London: Angus and Robertson, 1973.

DURKHEIM, E. *Suicide: A Study in Sociology.* New York: Free Press, 1951. (Originally published 1897.)

ENGEL, G. L. "The Psychosomatic Approach to Individual Susceptibility to Disease." *Gastroenterology,* 1974, *67,* 1085–1093.

ENGEL, G. L. "The Need for a New Medical Model: A Challenge for Biomedicine." *Science,* 1977, *196,* 129–136.

ENGEL, G. L., AND SCHMALE, A. H. "Conservation-Withdrawal: A Primary Regulatory Process for Organismic Homeostasis." In Ciba Foundation, *Physiology, Emotion, and Psychosomatic Illness.* Symposium 8. Amsterdam: Elsevier, 1972.

ERIKSON, E. H. "Growth and Crises of the 'Healthy Personality.'" In J. E. Senn (Ed.), *Symposium on the Healthy Personality.* New York: Josiah Macy, Jr., Foundation, 1950.

ERIKSON, E. H. "The Problem of Ego Identity." *Journal of the American Psychoanalytic Association,* 1956, *4,* 58–121. (Reprinted in M. R. Stein, A. J. Vidich, and D. M. White (Eds.), *Identity and Anxiety.* New York: Free Press, 1960.)

ERIKSON, E. H. *Young Man Luther: A Study in Psychoanalysis and History.* New York: Norton, 1958.

ERIKSON, E. H. "Identity, Psychosocial." In D. L. Sills (Ed.), *The International Encyclopedia of the Social Sciences.* Vol. 7. New York: Macmillan, 1968.

EYER, J., AND STERLING, P. "Stress-Related Mortality and Social Organization." *Review of Radical Political Economy,* 1977, *9,* 1–44.

FANSHEL, S. "A Meaningful Measure of Health for Epidemiology." *International Journal of Epidemiology,* 1972, *1,* 319–337.

FELDMAN, J. J. "The Household Interview Survey as a Technique for the Collection of Morbidity Data." *Journal of Chronic Diseases,* 1960, *11,* 535–557.

FRANK, J. D. "Mind-Body Relationships in Illness and Healing." *Preventive Medicine,* 1975, *2,* 46–59.

FRANKENHAUESER, M., AND GARDELL, B. "Underload and Overload

in Working Life: Outline of a Multidisciplinary Approach." *Journal of Human Stress*, 1976, *2* (3), 35–46.

FREIDSON, E. *Professional Dominance*. New York: Atherton, 1970.

FROMM, E. *Escape from Freedom*. New York: Holt, Rinehart and Winston, 1941.

GALDSTON, I. (Ed.). *Beyond the Germ Theory: The Roles of Deprivation and Stress in Health and Disease*. New York: Health Education Council, 1954.

GALLAGHER, E. B. (Ed.). *The Doctor-Patient Relationship in the Changing Health Scene*. DHEW Publication No. NIMH 78–183. Washington, D.C.: Public Health Service, 1978.

GARFIELD, S. R. "The Delivery of Medical Care." *Scientific American*, 1970, *222*, 15–23.

GARFIELD, S. R., AND OTHERS. "Evaluation of a New Ambulatory Medical Care Delivery System." *New England Journal of Medicine*, 1976, *294*, 426–431.

GLASS, D. C. "Stress, Behavior Patterns, and Coronary Disease." *American Scientist*, 1977, *65*, 177–187.

GOFFMAN, E. *Asylums*. New York: Doubleday, 1961.

GOVE, W. R. "Societal Reaction as an Explanation of Mental Illness." *American Sociological Review*, 1970, *35*, 873–884.

GOVE, W. R. "Sex, Marital Status, and Mortality." *American Journal of Sociology*, 1973, *79*, 45–67.

GUNDERSON, E. K. E., AND RAHE, R. H. (Eds.). *Life Stress and Illness*. Springfield, Ill.: Thomas, 1974.

GUTMAN, H. G. *The Black Family in Slavery and Freedom*. New York: Pantheon, 1976.

GUTTMAN, L. "Measurement as Structural Theory." *Psychometrika*, 1974, *36*, 329–347.

HINKLE, L. E., JR. "The Effect of Exposure to Culture Change, Social Change, and Changes in Interpersonal Relationships on Health." In B. Dohrenwend and B. Dohrenwend (Eds.), *Stressful Life Events: Their Nature and Effects*. New York: Wiley, 1974.

HINKLE, L. E., JR. "Measurement of the Effects of the Environment upon the Health and Behavior of People." In L. E. Hinkle, Jr., and W. C. Loring (Eds.), *The Effect of the Man-Made Environ-*

ment on Health and Behavior. Atlanta: Center for Disease Control, Public Health Service, 1977.

HINKLE, L. E., JR., AND LORING, W. C. (Eds.)'. *The Effect of the Man-Made Environment on Health and Behavior.* Atlanta: Center for Disease Control, Public Health Service, 1977.

HINKLE, L. E., JR., AND WOLFF, H. G. "Health and Social Environment: Experimental Investigations." In A. Leighton and others (Eds.), *Explorations in Social Psychiatry.* New York: Basic Books, 1957.

HOCHSCHILD, A. R. "Disengagement Theory: A Critique and Proposal." *American Sociological Review,* 1975, *40,* 553–569.

HOLMES, O. W. *The Autocrat of the Breakfast-Table.* (Rev. ed.) Boston: Houghton Mifflin, 1884.

HOLMES, T. H., AND MASUDA, M. "Life Change and Illness Susceptibility." In B. Dohrenwend and B. Dohrenwend (Eds.), *Stressful Life Events: Their Nature and Effects.* New York: Wiley, 1974.

HOLMES, T. H., AND RAHE, R. H. "The Social Readjustment Rating Scale." *Journal of Psychosomatic Research,* 1967, *11,* 213–218.

ILLICH, I. *Tools for Conviviality.* New York: Harper & Row, 1973.

ILLICH, I. *Medical Nemesis: The Expropriation of Health.* New York: Bantam, 1976.

JACOBS, S., AND OSTFELD, A. "An Epidemiological Review of the Mortality of Bereavement." *Psychosomatic Medicine,* 1977, *39,* 344–357.

JONES, E. *The Life and Work of Sigmund Freud.* (Edited and abridged in one volume by L. Trilling and S. Marcus.) New York: Basic Books, 1961.

JUSTICE, B., AND DUNCAN, D. F. "Life Crises as a Precursor to Child Abuse." *Public Health Reports,* 1976, *91,* 110–115.

KAGAN, A. R., AND LEVI, L. "Health and Environment. Psychosocial Stimuli: A Review." *Social Science and Medicine,* 1974, *8,* 225–241.

KANTER, R. M. "Commitment and Social Organization." *American Sociological Review,* 1968, *33,* 499–517.

KAPLAN, B. H., CASSEL, J. C., AND GORE, S. "Social Support and Health." *Medical Care,* 1977, *25* (suppl.), 47–58.

KARDINER, A. *The Individual and His Society.* New York: Columbia University Press, 1939.

KARDINER, A. *The Psychological Frontiers of Society.* New York: Columbia University Press, 1945.

KARDINER, A., AND OVESEY, L. *The Mark of Oppression.* New York: World, 1951.

KASL, S. V. "The Effects of the Residential Environment on Health and Behavior: A Review." In L. E. Hinkle, Jr., and W. C. Loring (Eds.), *The Effect of the Man-Made Environment on Health and Behavior.* Atlanta: Center for Disease Control, Public Health Service, 1977.

KIRITZ, S., AND MOOS, R. H. "Physiological Effects of the Social Environment." In P. M. Insel and R. H. Moos (Eds.), *Health and the Social Environment.* Lexington, Mass.: Heath, 1974.

KLEINMAN, A., EISENBERG, L., AND GOOD, B. "Culture, Illness and Care: Clinical Lessons from Anthropological and Cross-Cultural Research." *Annals of Internal Medicine,* 1978, *88,* 251–258.

KNUPFER, G. "Portrait of the Underdog." *Public Opinion Quarterly,* 1947, *11,* 103–114.

KOHN, M. L. "Social Class and Schizophrenia: A Critical Review." In D. Rosenthal and S. S. Kety (Eds.), *The Transmission of Schizophrenia.* Oxford: Pergamon Press, 1968.

KOHN, M. L. *Class and Conformity: A Study in Values.* (1st ed.) Homewood, Ill.: Dorsey Press, 1969.

KOHN, M. L. "Social Class and Schizophrenia: A Critical Review and a Reformulation." *Schizophrenia Bulletin,* 1973, *7,* 60–79.

KOHN, M. L. "The Interaction of Social Class and Other Factors in the Etiology of Schizophrenia." *American Journal of Psychiatry,* 1976a, *133,* 177–180.

KOHN, M. L. "Occupational Structure and Alienation." *American Journal of Sociology,* 1976b, *82,* 111–130.

KOHN, M. L. "The Substantive Complexity of Work and Its Relationship to Adult Personality." In E. H. Erikson and N. Smelser (Eds.), forthcoming.

KOHN, M. L., AND SCHOOLER, C. "The Reciprocal Effects of the Substantive Complexity of Work and Intellectual Flexibility: A Longitudinal Assessment." *American Journal of Sociology,* 1978, *84,* 24–52.

KOSA, J., ANTONOVSKY, A., AND ZOLA, I. K. (Eds.). *Poverty and*

Health: A Sociological Analysis. Cambridge, Mass.: Harvard University Press, 1969.

KUHN, T. *The Structure of Scientific Revolutions.* Chicago: University of Chicago Press, 1962.

LAZARUS, R. S., AND COHEN, J. B. "Environmental Stress." In I. Altman and J. F. Wohlwill (Eds.), *Human Behavior and Environment.* Vol. 2. New York: Plenum, 1977.

LEFCOURT, H. M. *Locus of Control: Current Trends in Theory and Research.* New York: Wiley, 1976.

LERNER, I. M. *Heredity, Evolution and Society.* San Francisco: W. H. Freeman, 1968.

LESHAN, L. *You Can Fight for Your Life: Emotional Factors in the Causation of Cancer.* New York: Harcourt Brace Jovanovich, 1978.

LEVI, L. "Psychosocial Stress and Disease: A Conceptual Model." In E. K. E. Gunderson and R. H. Rahe (Eds.), *Life Stress and Illness.* Springfield, Ill.: Thomas, 1974.

LEVIN, D. L., AND OTHERS. *Cancer Rates and Risks.* (2nd ed.) Washington, D.C.: Public Health Service, 1974.

LEWIS, C. E., AND LEWIS, M. A. "The Potential Impact of Sexual Equality on Health." *New England Journal of Medicine,* 1977, *297,* 863–869.

LEWIS, O. "The Culture of Poverty," *Anthropological Essays.* New York: Random House, 1970.

LIDDELL, H. S. "Sheep and Goats: The Psychological Effects of Laboratory Experiences of Deprivation and Stress upon Certain Experimental Animals." In I. Galdston (Ed.), *Beyond the Germ Theory.* New York: Health Education Council, 1954.

LOWENTHAL, M. F., AND CHIRIBOGA, D. "Social Stress and Adaptation: Toward a Life Course Perspective." In C. Eisdorfer and M. P. Lawton (Eds.), *The Psychology of Adult Development and Aging.* Washington, D.C.: American Psychological Association, 1973.

MC ALPINE, D., LUMSDEN, C. E., AND ACHESON, E. D. *Multiple Sclerosis: A Reappraisal.* (2nd ed.) Edinburgh and London: Churchill Livingstone, 1972.

MC KEOWN, T. *The Role of Medicine: Dream, Mirage, or Nemesis?* London: Nuffield Provincial Hospitals Trust, 1976.

MC KINLAY, J. B. "The Changing Political and Economic Context of the Patient-Physician Encounter." In E. B. Gallagher (Ed.), *The Doctor-Patient Relationship in the Changing Health Scene.* Washington, D.C.: Public Health Service, 1978.

MALINOWSKI, B. "Culture." In E. R. A. Seligman (Ed.), *The Encyclopedia of the Social Sciences.* Vol. 4. New York: Macmillan, 1931.

MAOZ, B., AND OTHERS. "Female Attitudes to Menopause." *Social Psychiatry,* 1970, *5,* 35–40.

MATHEWS, K. A., AND OTHERS. "Competitive Drive, Pattern A, and Coronary Heart Disease: A Further Analysis of Some Data from the Western Collaborative Group Study." *Journal of Chronic Diseases,* 1977, *30,* 489–498.

MECHANIC, D. *Students Under Stress: A Study in the Social Psychology of Adaptation.* New York: Free Press, 1962.

MECHANIC, D. *Medical Sociology: A Selective View.* New York: Free Press, 1968.

MEDAWAR, P. "Review of L. Leshan's *You Can Fight for Your Life.*" *New York Review of Books,* June 9, 1977.

MERCER, J. R. "Who Is Normal? Two Perspectives on Mild Mental Retardation." In E. G. Jaco (Ed.), *Patients, Physicians and Illness.* (2nd ed.) New York: Free Press, 1972.

MERTON, R. K. "Social Structure and Anomie," *Social Theory and Social Structure.* New York: Free Press, 1957.

MERTON, R. K. *Social Theory and Social Structure.* (Expanded ed.) New York: Free Press, 1968.

MERTON, R. K. "The Ambivalence of Physicians," *Sociological Ambivalence and Other Essays.* New York: Free Press, 1976.

MONJAN, A. A., AND COLLECTOR, M. I. "Stress-Induced Modulation of the Immune Response." *Science,* 1977, *196,* 307–308.

MORRIS, J. N. *Uses of Epidemiology.* Edinburgh and London: Churchill Livingstone, 1957.

MOSS, G. E. *Illness, Immunity and Social Interaction: The Dynamics of Biosocial Resonation.* New York: Wiley, 1973.

NADITCH, M. P. "Locus of Control, Relative Discontent and Hypertension." *Social Psychiatry,* 1974, *9,* 111–117.

National Center for Health Statistics. "Prevalence of Selected

Chronic Digestive Conditions, United States, July-December, 1968." *Vital and Health Statistics,* 1973a, Series 10, No. 83.

National Center for Health Statistics. "Prevalence of Selected Chronic Respiratory Conditions, United States, 1970." *Vital and Health Statistics,* 1973b, Series 10, No. 84.

National Center for Health Statistics. "Prevalence of Chronic Circulatory Conditions, United States, 1972." *Vital and Health Statistics,* 1974, Series 10, No. 94.

National Center for Health Statistics. "Prevalence of Selected Impairments, United States, 1971." *Vital and Health Statistics,* 1975, Series 10, No. 99.

National Center for Health Statistics. *Health: United States, 1975.* DHEW Publication No. HRA 76-1232. Rockville, Md.: Department of Health, Education, and Welfare, 1976.

National Center for Health Statistics. "Current Estimates from the Health Interview Survey, United States, 1976." *Vital and Health Statistics,* 1977a, Series 10, No. 119.

National Center for Health Statistics. "Profile of Chronic Illness in Nursing Homes, United States: National Nursing Home Survey." *Vital and Health Statistics,* 1977b, Series 13, No. 29.

National Center for Health Statistics. "Acute Conditions, Incidence, and Associated Disability, United States, July 1975–June 1976." *Vital and Health Statistics,* 1978, Series 10, No. 120.

National Health Education Committee. *The Killers and the Cripplers: Facts on Major Diseases in the United States Today.* New York: McKay, 1976.

NISBET, R. *The Social Philosophers: Community and Conflict in Western Thought.* New York: Crowell, 1973.

NUCKOLLS, K. B., CASSEL, J., AND KAPLAN, B. H. "Psychosocial Assets, Life Crisis and the Prognosis of Pregnancy." *American Journal of Epidemiology,* 1972, 95, 431–441.

OAKLEY, A. *Woman's Work.* New York: Pantheon, 1975.

OBEYESEKERE, G. "Psycho-Cultural Exegesis of a Case of Spirit Possession from Sri Lanka." *Contributions to Asian Studies,* 1973, 8, 41–89.

OETTGEN, H. F. "Immunotherapy of Cancer." *New England Journal of Medicine,* 1977, 297, 484–491.

OSTFELD, A. M., AND D'ATRI, D. A. "Psychophysiological Responses to the Urban Environment." *International Journal of Psychiatry in Medicine*, 1975, *6*, 15–28.

PARKES, C. M. "Psychosocial Transitions: A Field for Study." *Social Science and Medicine*, 1971, *5*, 101–115.

PARKES, C. M. *Bereavement: Studies of Grief in Adult Life*. New York: International Universities Press, 1972.

PARKES, C. M., BENJAMIN, B., AND FITZGERALD, R. G. "Broken Heart: A Statistical Study of Increased Mortality Among Widowers." *British Medical Journal*, 1969, *1*, 740–743.

PARSONS, T. *The Social System*. New York: Free Press, 1951.

PARSONS, T. "Epilogue." In E. B. Gallagher (Ed.), *The Doctor-Patient Relationship in the Changing Health Scene*. DHEW Publication No. NIMH 78-183. Washington, D.C.: Public Health Service, 1978.

PEARLIN, L. I. "Sex Roles and Depression." In N. Datan and L. H. Ginsberg (Eds.), *Normative Life Crises*. New York: Academic Press, 1975.

PEARLIN, L. I., AND JOHNSON, J. S. "Marital Status, Life-Strains and Depression." *American Sociological Review*, 1977, *42*, 704–715.

PEARLIN, L. I., AND SCHOOLER, C. "The Structure of Coping." *Journal of Health and Social Behavior*, 1978, *19*, 2–21.

PERLMUTER, L. C., AND MONTY, R. A. "The Importance of Perceived Control: Fact or Fantasy?" *American Scientist*, 1977, *65*, 759–765.

PETRIE, A. *Individuality in Pain and Suffering*. Chicago: University of Chicago Press, 1967.

PHILLIPS, D. P., AND FELDMAN, K. A. "A Dip in Deaths Before Ceremonial Occasions: Some New Relationships Between Social Integration and Mortality." *American Sociological Review*, 1973, *38*, 678–696.

POWLES, J. "On the Limitations of Modern Medicine." *Science, Medicine and Man*, 1973, *1*, 1–30.

RADLOFF, R., AND HELMREICH, R. *Groups Under Stress: Psychological Research in SEALAB II*. New York: Appleton-Century-Crofts, 1968.

RAHE, R. H. "The Pathway Between Subjects' Recent Life Changes and Their Near-Future Illness Reports." In B. Dohrenwend and

B. Dohrenwend (Eds.), *Stressful Life Events: Their Nature and Effects.* New York: Wiley, 1974.

RAHE, R. H. "Editorial: Life Change Measurement Clarification." *Psychosomatic Medicine,* 1978, *40,* 95–98.

RAPOPORT, A. "The Promise and Pitfalls of Information Theory." In W. Buckley (Ed.), *Modern Systems Research for the Behavioral Scientist.* Chicago: Aldine, 1968.

ROAZEN, P. *Freud: Political and Social Thought.* New York: Knopf, 1968.

ROESKE, N. A. "The Emotional Response to Hysterectomy." *Psychiatric Opinion,* 1978, *15* (2), 11–20.

ROSENSTOCK, I. M. "What Research in Motivation Suggests for Public Health." *American Journal of Public Health,* 1960, *50,* 295–302.

ROTTER, J. B. *Generalized Expectancies for Internal Versus External Control of Reinforcement.* Psychological Monographs No. 80, 1966.

ROUECHE, B. "Annals of Medicine: Antipathies." *New Yorker,* March 13, 1978, pp. 61–84.

RUESCH, J. *Duodenal Ulcer.* Berkeley: University of California Press, 1948.

RUTSTEIN, D. D., AND OTHERS. "Measuring the Quality of Medical Care." *New England Journal of Medicine,* 1976, *294,* 582–588.

SCHACHTEL, E. G. "On Alienated Concepts of Identity." In E. Josephson and M. Josephson (Eds.), *Man Alone.* New York: Dell, 1962.

SCHEFF, T. J. *Being Mentally Ill.* Chicago: Aldine, 1966.

SCHMALE, A. H. "Giving Up as a Final Common Pathway to Changes in Health." In Z. J. Lipowski (Ed.), *Advances in Psychosomatic Medicine.* Vol. 8. Basel, Switzerland: S. Karger, 1972.

SCHRÖDINGER, E. "Quote from *What Is Life?*" In W. Buckley (Ed.), *Modern Systems Research for the Behavioral Scientist.* Chicago: Aldine, 1968.

SCHUR, M. *Freud: Living and Dying.* New York: International Universities Press, 1972.

SCOTT, R. A. *The Making of Blind Men: A Study of Adult Socialization.* New York: Russell Sage Foundation, 1969.

SCOTT, R. A., AND HOWARD, A. "Models of Stress." In S. Levine and N. A. Scotch (Eds.), *Social Stress*. Chicago: Aldine, 1970.

SELIGMAN, M. E. P. *Helplessness: On Depression, Development, and Death*. San Francisco: W. H. Freeman, 1975.

SELYE, H. *The Stress of Life*. New York: McGraw-Hill, 1956.

SELYE, H. "Confusion and Controversy in the Stress Field." *Journal of Human Stress*, 1975, *1*, 37–44.

SHALIT, B. "Structural Ambiguity and Limits to Coping." *Journal of Human Stress*, 1977, *3* (4), 32–45.

SHEEHY, G. *Passages: Predictable Crises of Adult Life*. New York: Dutton, 1974.

SHUVAL, J. T. "Some Persistent Effects of Trauma: Five Years After the Nazi Concentration Camps." *Social Problems*, 1957–1958, *5*, 230–243.

SHUVAL, J. T., ANTONOVSKY, A., AND DAVIES, A. M. *Social Functions of Medical Practice: Doctor-Patient Relationships in Israel*. San Francisco: Jossey-Bass, 1970.

SIMMEL, G. *Conflict and the Web of Group Affiliations*. (K. H. Wolff and R. Bendix, Trans.) New York: Free Press, 1955.

SIMON, W., AND GAGNON, J. H. "The Anomie of Affluence: A Post-Mertonian Conception." *American Journal of Sociology*, 1976, *82*, 356–378.

SOLOMON, G. F., AND AMKRAUT, A. A. "Emotions, Stress and Immunity." In P. M. Insel and R. H. Moos (Eds.), *Health and the Social Environment*. Lexington, Mass.: Heath, 1974.

SOROCHAN, W. D. "Health Concepts as a Basis for Orthobiosis." In E. Hart and W. Sechrist (Eds.), *Dynamics of Wellness*. Belmont, Calif.: Wadsworth, 1970.

SROLE, L., AND OTHERS. *Mental Health in the Metropolis: The Midtown Study*. Vol. 1. New York: McGraw-Hill, 1962.

STARR, P. "Review of W. Gaylin and others' *The Limits of Benevolence*." *New York Times Book Review*, May 21, 1978, p. 9.

SUSSER, M. *Community Psychiatry: Epidemiologic and Social Themes*. New York: Random House, 1968.

SUSSER, M. "Ethical Components in the Definition of Health." *International Journal of Health Services*, 1974, *4*, 539–548.

SWEENEY, D. R., TINLING, D. C., AND SCHMALE, A. H., JR. "Differentiation of the 'Giving Up' Affects—Helplessness and Hopelessness." *Archives of General Psychiatry*, 1970, *23*, 378–382.

SYME, S. L., AND BERKMAN, L. F. "Social Class, Susceptibility, and Sickness." *American Journal of Epidemiology,* 1976, *104,* 1–8.

SYME, S. L., AND TORFS, C. P. "Epidemiologic Research in Hypertension: A Critical Appraisal." *Journal of Human Stress,* 1978, *4,* 43–48.

SZASZ, T. *The Myth of Mental Illness.* New York: Hoeber Harper, 1963.

SZASZ, T., AND HOLLENDER, M. H. "A Contribution to the Philosophy of Medicine: The Basic Models of the Doctor-Patient Relationship." *Archives of Internal Medicine,* 1956, *97,* 585–592.

TAEUBER, C. (Ed.). *America in the Seventies: Some Social Indicators.* Philadelphia: American Academy of Political and Social Sciences, 1978.

THACKER, S. B., GREEN, S. B., AND SALBER, E. J. "Hospitalizations in a Southern Rural Community: An Application of the 'Ecology Model.' " *International Journal of Epidemiology,* 1977, *6,* 55–63.

THOMAS, L. *The Lives of a Cell.* Toronto: Bantam Books of Canada, 1974.

TOFFLER, A. *Future Shock.* New York: Random House, 1970.

TYROLER, H. A., AND CASSEL, J. C. "Health Consequences of Culture Change: The Effect of Urbanization on Coronary Heart Mortality in Rural Residents of North Carolina." *Journal of Chronic Diseases,* 1964, *17,* 167–177.

VICKERS, G. "The Concept of Stress in Relation to the Disorganization of Human Behavior." In W. Buckley (Ed.), *Modern Systems Research for the Behavioral Scientist.* Chicago: Aldine, 1968.

WEISENBERG, M. "Pain and Pain Control." *Psychological Bulletin,* 1977, *84,* 1008–1044.

WEISSMAN, M. M., AND PAYKEL, E. S. "Moving and Depression in Women." *Transaction/SOCIETY,* 1972, *9* (9), 24–28.

WERTHEIM, E. S. "Positive Mental Health, Western Society and the Family." *International Journal of Social Psychiatry,* 1974, *21,* 982/1–5.

WERTHEIM, E. S. "Person-Environment Interaction: The Epigenesis of Autonomy and Competence." *British Journal of Medical Psychology,* 1975, *48,* 1–8, 95–111, 237–256, 391–402.

WERTHEIM, E. S. "Developmental Genesis of Human Vulnerability:

Conceptual Re-Evaluation." In J. E. Anthony and E. Koupernik (Eds.), *Vulnerable Children.* Yearbook of the International Association for Child Psychiatry and Allied Professions, Vol. 4. New York: Wiley, 1978.

WHITE, K. L., WILLIAMS, T. F., AND GREENBERG, B. G. "The Ecology of Medical Care." *New England Journal of Medicine,* 1961, *265,* 885.

WINKELSTEIN, W. "Epidemiological Considerations Underlying the Allocation of Health and Disease Care Resources." *International Journal of Epidemiology,* 1972, *1,* 69–74.

WOHLWILL, J. F. "The Physical Environment: A Problem for a Psychology of Stimulation." In H. C. Lindgren and others (Eds.), *Current Research in Psychology.* New York: Wiley, 1971.

WOLF, S., AND GOODELL, H. *Harold G. Wolff's Stress and Disease.* (2nd ed.) Springfield, Ill.: Thomas, 1968.

YOUNG, A. "Internalizing and Externalizing Medical Belief Systems: An Ethiopian Example." *Social Science and Medicine,* 1976a, *10,* 147–156.

YOUNG, A. "Some Implications of Medical Beliefs and Practices for Social Anthropology." *American Anthropologist,* 1976b, *78,* 5–24.

YOUNG, A. "Order, Analogy and Efficacy in Ethiopian Medical Divination." *Culture, Medicine and Psychiatry,* 1977, *1,* 183–199.

ZOLA, I. K. "Culture and Symptoms: An Analysis of Patients' Presenting Complaints." *American Sociological Review,* 1966, *31,* 615–630.

Index

A

Accidents and survivors, as psycho-social stressor, 80–81
ACHESON, E. D., 34, 239
Action implication: as breakdown facet, 62–64; concept of, 63
Acute morbidity condition: defined, 28; prevalence of, 27–28, 29
Aggression, as psychosocial stressor, 82
Alcohol abuse, data on, 22
ALEXANDER, F., 105, 229
Allergy, data on, 19, 20, 22, 26
Alorese culture, and sense of coherence, 150
American Cancer Society, 23
AMKRAUT, A. A., 181, 244
ANDREWS, F. M., 68, 229
Anemia, data on, 19
Animal studies, and health linked to sense of coherence, 179
ANTONOVSKY, A., 2, 3, 4, 5, 6, 43, 56, 62, 64, 68, 69, 74, 77, 93, 96, 99, 101, 106, 108, 115, 116, 117, 153, 162, 163, 217, 229–231, 234, 238–239, 244
ANTONOVSKY, H., 116, 117, 231
ARIAN, A., 68, 230
Arthritis, data on, 22
Artifactual-material factors, as generalized resistance resources, 106–107
Autonomy, sense of coherence related to, 140–141

B

BAHNSON, C. B., 173, 231
BECKER, E., 82, 231
BECKER, H., 25, 231
BELLOC, N. B., 31, 54–55, 231
BENJAMIN, B., 189, 242
BEN-SIRA, Z., 207, 231
BENSMAN, J., 156, 231

247

Bereavement, and health linked to sense of coherence, 166
BERKMAN, L. F., 66, 115, 163–165, 168, 231, 245
BERNSTEIN, J., 3, 108, 163, 230
Bias, cultural, danger of, 152–158
Biochemical factors, as generalized resistance resources, 103–106
Birth defects, data on, 21
BLUM, H. L., 18–19, 24, 231–232
BOOTH, A., 178, 232
BOWLBY, J., 139, 232
Breakdown: concept of, 4–5; continuum of, 55–64; mapping sentence of, 64–65; and negative life events, 177; profile of, 64–67
BRESLOW, L., 31, 54–55, 59, 231, 232
BRIDGES-WEBB, C., 16, 232
BRINTON, C., 134–136, 157, 232
Bronchitis, chronic, data on, 19, 22
BRONFENBRENNER, U., 85, 87, 232
BUCKLEY, W., 78, 232
Bureaucratic modality, of doctor-patient relationship, 209, 210, 213–214, 215
BURNET, M., 14, 78–79, 103, 220, 232
BUTLER, S., 102

C

Cancer, psychological factors in, 173
CANNON, W. B., 71, 129, 165, 176, 232
CAPLOVITZ, D., 108, 232
Cardiovascular diseases, data on, 19
CAROLINE, N. L., 193n, 232
CASSEL, J. C., 83, 166–167, 168, 171, 178–179, 180, 232–233, 237, 241, 245
CASSELL, E. J., 36–37, 43–44, 204–206, 211–212, 213, 233
Cataclysmic events, as stressors, 74, 80, 87, 188
Center for Disease Control, 26, 27n, 233
CHAN, K. B., 122, 233
Change: and health linked to sense of coherence, 169–171, 189; as psychosocial stressor, 83
Childrearing: in salutogenic model,

187, 191; sense of coherence related to, 139–142, 146–147
CHIRIBOGA, D., 114, 239
Chronic conditions, substantial, defined, 18
Circulatory conditions, chronic, data on, 23
Clearinghouse on Health Indices, 50n
COBB, S., 115, 168, 233
COCHRANE, A. L., 47–48, 101, 233
Cognitive appraisal, coping related to, 111
Cognitive factors, as generalized resistance resources, 107–110
COHEN, J. B., 72, 74, 80, 87, 111, 239
Coherence, sense of: case histories of, 128–136; continuum for, 158; and cultural bias, 156–158; defined, 123–128; direct evidence of link with health by, 161–163; ego identity distinct from, 109–110; emergence of, 187–188; evolution of perspective on, 1–11; fake, 158–159; and generalized resistance resources, 122; global orientation of, 180; and health care system, 198–219; and health outlook, 220–227; health related to, 160–181; indirect evidence of link with health by, 163–179; modification of, 188; operationalizing, 158–159; perceptions of, 123–159; in salutogenic model, 183, 186–187; sources of, 136–152, 190–192
COLLECTOR, M. I., 96, 240
Collegial modality, of doctor-patient relationship, 208, 209, 211–212, 215
COLLEN, M. F., 31–32, 233
Comanche culture, and sense of coherence, 150
Commission on Chronic Illness, 17–22, 233–234
Commitment, concept of, 116–117
Competence, sense of coherence related to, 140–141
Complexity: sense of coherence related to, 148; substantive, of work, 144–145, 147, 148

Conformity/self-direction, sense of coherence related to, 144, 146–147

Conservation-withdrawal, sense of coherence related to, 138–139, 166

Consistency, sense of coherence related to, 187, 189, 200, 208

Control: locus of, 152–154, 158, 171–172; personal, 154–155; sense of, related to sense of coherence, 127–128

Coping: ability for, 162–163; concept of, 110–111, 112; functions of, 194; as generalized resistance resource, 110–114; sex differences in, 148

Coronary heart disease, and Type A behavior pattern, 174–175

COSER, L., 157, 234

COSER, R. L., 137, 145–149, 234

COUSINS, N., 128–132, 195, 234

COWELL, J., 178, 232

CROSSMAN, R., 127, 234

Crowding, and health linked to sense of coherence, 178–179

Cultural-historical sources, for sense of coherence, 149–152

Cultural variables, and health linked to sense of coherence, 168–171

CUTLER, S. J., 23, 234

D

D'ATRI, D. A., 169, 241–242

DAHRENDORF, R., 88, 234

DATAN, N., 6, 86, 115, 234

DAVIES, A. M., 2, 43, 244

Deafness, data on, 18, 20–21

Democratic modality, of doctor-patient relationship, 209, 210–211, 214

Dental caries, data on, 24–25

Depression, helplessness related to, 172

Destruction, as psychosocial stressor, 82

Diabetes, data on, 18, 22

Digestive diseases, data on, 21, 24

Disability: causes of, 22; prevalence of, 28, 30

Dis-ease, concept of, 5

Disease: illness distinct from, 43, 204–206; notifiable, prevalence of, 26–27

Disease care system: clinical model of, 39–45; number of people in, 42; public health model of, 45–47. *See also* Health care system

DOBZHANSKY, T., 104, 234

DODGE, D. L., 166, 168, 234

DOHRENWEND, B., 176, 177, 234

DOHRENWEND, B., 176, 177, 234

DORN, H. F., 23, 234

DOSTOEVSKY, F., 124

Drive reduction, tension related to, 95–96

DUBOS, R. J., 5, 11, 13, 16, 53, 79, 104, 105, 193, 221, 222–223, 224, 225, 226, 234–235

DUNCAN, D. F., 143, 237

DURKHEIM, E., 91, 235

Dynamic, related to sense of coherence, 125

E

Ego identity: in salutogenic model, 187–188, 191; sense of coherence distinct from, 109–110; and tension management, 108–110

EISENBERG, L., 43, 212, 238

Emotional affect, and coping strategies, 114

Emotional factors, as generalized resistance resources, 107–110

Emphysema, pulmonary, data on, 19

ENGEL, G. L., 107, 137, 138, 139, 141, 152, 162, 166, 173, 179, 235

Entropy: negative, and generalized resistance resources, 120–122; stressors related to, 77–78

Epidemiology, and health care, 45–47

ERIKSON, E. H., 85, 109, 151, 235

Expectant faith, and health linked to sense of coherence, 172–173

EYER, J., 39n, 235

F

Facet theory, and breakdown, 57

FANSHEL, S., 47, 50–51, 59, 235
Farsightedness, as coping strategy, 113, 170
FELDMAN, J. J., 23, 235
FELDMAN, K. A., 114, 242
FITZGERALD, R. G., 189, 242
Flexibility, as coping strategy, 113, 170
FLEXNER, A., 214
FOX, R., 82
FRANK, J. D., 172–173, 235
FRANKENHAUESER, M., 87, 148, 235–236
FREIDSON, E., 213, 236
FREUD, S., 81–82, 132–134, 195
FRIED, M., 3
FRIEDMAN, M., 173–174
FROMM, E., 151, 236
Functional limitation: as breakdown facet, 59–61; concept of, 60
Functioning, concept of, 50

G

GAGNON, J. H., 88–89, 244
GALDSTON, I., 80, 87, 236
GALLAGHER, E. B., 214, 236
GARDELL, B., 87, 148, 235–236
GARFIELD, S. R., 46, 236
GAYLIN, W., 218
Generalized resistance resources (GRRs): absence of, as stressor, 119–120; analysis of, 102–119; concept of, 5, 99; dual function of, 194–195; general adaptation syndrome distinct from, 105; mapping sentence of, 102–103, 120–121; meaning of, 99–100; as negative entropy providers, 120–122; in salutogenic model, 189–192; significance of, 122; sources of, 137, 152, 190–192; and tension management, 98–122
Genetics, stressors related to, 78–79
GINSBERG, L. H., 86, 234
Giving-up syndrome, sense of coherence related to, 137–138, 162
GLASS, D. C., 175, 180, 236
Goal achievement, as psychosocial stressor, 88–89

GOFFMAN, E., 25, 149n, 236
GOOD, B., 43, 212, 238
GOODELL, H., 75–76, 105, 169, 170, 246
GORE, S., 166, 167, 237
GOVE, W. R., 25, 114, 165, 236
GREEN, S. B., 42, 245
GREENBERG, B. G., 16–17, 246
Group Health Insurance, 43
GUNDERSON, E. K. E., 176, 236
GUTMAN, H. G., 8, 236
GUTTMAN, L., 8, 57, 236

H

HARTMAN, H., 101, 230
Health: clinical model of, 39–45; as a continuum, 38–69; continuum model of, 47–52; defined, 52, 53; dichotomous model of, implications of, 43–45; outlook for, 220–227; in salutogenic model, 196–197; salutogenic model of, 182–197; sense of coherence related to, 160–181; study of, rather than disease, 12–37; and value systems, 48–50
Health care: availability of, 217; preventive, 217–218
Health care system: and high-risk groups, 218–219; implications of sense of coherence for, 198–219; modalities of relationships in, 207–214; patients in relationship with, 199–214; routine encounters in, 202–207; and social structure, 214–219; traumatic situations in, 200–202; trust in practitioners of, 218. See also Disease care system
Health ease/dis-ease. See Breakdown
Health Insurance Plan, 43
HELMREICH, R., 95, 242
Helplessness: depression related to, 172; sense of coherence related to, 138, 139–140; and Type A behavior, 175
HINKLE, L. E., JR., 76, 79, 169, 170–171, 236–237
Historical sources, for sense of coherence, 149–152

History: horrors of, as psychosocial stressor, 82; immediacy of, as psychosocial stressor, 83
HOCHSCHILD, A. R., 114–115, 237
HOCHSTIM, J. R., 31, 54–55, 231
HOLLENDER, M. H., 205, 245
HOLMES, O. W., 83–84, 195, 237
HOLMES, T. H., 75, 81, 86, 93–94, 143, 176–177, 237
Homeostasis, stressors related to, 71–72, 80
Hopelessness, sense of coherence related to, 138
HOWARD, A., 72, 112, 244
Human Ecology Study Program, 75–76, 170, 176
Hyperuricemia, data on, 19

I

ILLICH, I., 11, 203, 221, 223–224, 225, 226, 237
Illness: chronic, prevalence of, 17–26; disease distinct from, 43, 204–206
Immunological surveillance, concept of, 103
Immunopotentiators, and tension management, 104
Intelligence, and tension management, 107–108
Interpersonal-relational factors, as generalized resistance resources, 114–117
Intrapsychic conflict, as psychosocial stressor, 81–82

J

JACOBS, S., 166, 237
JENKINS, D., 171, 233
JOHNSON, J. S., 172, 242
JONES, E., 132n, 237
JUSTICE, B., 143, 237

K

KAFKA, F., 127
KAGAN, A. R., 180, 237

Kaiser-Permanente, 31–32, 43, 46
KANTER, R. M., 116, 237
KAPLAN, B., 166, 167, 237, 241
KARDINER, A., 137, 149–152, 237–238
KASL, S. V., 169, 238
KATS, R., 2, 4, 74, 101, 230
KERANEN, G. M., 18–19, 24, 231–232
KIRITZ, S., 168, 238
KLEINMAN, A., 43, 212, 238
Knowledge-intelligence, and tension management, 107–108
KNUPFER, G., 108, 238
KOHN, M. L., 107, 137, 142–149, 161–162, 238
KOSA, J., 3, 77, 238–239
KUHN, T., 38, 239

L

Lawfulness, related to sense of coherence, 127
LAZARUS, R. S., 72, 73, 74, 80, 87, 110, 111, 239
LEFCOURT, H. M., 152, 158–159, 171, 239
LERNER, I. M., 104, 239
LESHAN, L., 173, 239
LEVI, L., 180, 237, 239
LEVIN, D. L., 23, 239
LEWIS, C. E., 156–157, 239
LEWIS, M. A., 156–157, 239
LEWIS, O., 143, 239
LIDDELL, H. S., 179, 239
Life cycle crises, normative, as psychosocial stressors, 84–86
Life events: and health linked to sense of coherence, 176–179; in salutogenic model, 187–189
Limitation: functional, as breakdown facet, 59–61; prevalence of, 28, 30
Load balance: and psychosocial stressors, 86–87, 95; sense of coherence related to, 187, 189, 200, 205, 208, 211, 216
Locus-of-control concept, sense of coherence related to, 152–154, 158, 171–172
LORING, W. C., 169, 237
LORWIN, L., 2, 230

LOWENTHAL, M. F., 114, 239
LUMSDEN, C. E., 34, 239

M

MC ALPINE, D., 34, 239
MC KEOWN, T., 11, 33, 39n, 101, 102, 221, 222, 223, 224–225, 226, 239
MC KINLAY, J. B., 210, 214, 240
Macrosociocultural factors, as generalized resistance resources, 117–119
Magic, and tension management, 118
MALINOWSKI, B., 117–118, 126, 240
MALRAUX, A., 80
MANN, T., 124
MAOZ, B., 6, 85, 115, 234, 240
Marital status, and health linked to sense of coherence, 165
Market modality, of doctor-patient relationship, 209–210, 215
MARTIN, W. T., 166, 168, 234
MASUDA, M., 75, 93–94, 176–177, 237
MATHEWS, K. A., 174, 240
MECHANIC, D., 94, 95, 101, 113, 240
MEDAWAR, P., 173, 240
Medical education, and modalities of relationships, 214–215
Medicine, technological levels of, 221–222. See also Health care system
Menopause: as psychosocial stressor, 84–85; and social supports, 115–116
Mental illness, data on, 25–26
Mental retardation, data on, 19, 25
MERCER, J. R., 49, 240
MERTON, R. K., 88–89, 119, 203, 240
MEYER, A., 176
Mobility, as stressor, 94–95
Modalities, impact of, on sense of coherence, 207–214
MONJAN, A. A., 96, 240
MONTY, R. A., 152–153, 242
MOOS, R. H., 168, 238
Morbidity: data on, 16–35; hypothesis of, 15–16; methodological issues in, 32–35; overall, 30–32
MORRIS, J. N., 4, 15, 240

MOSS, G. E., 72, 240
Mutilation, as psychosocial stressor, 82

N

NADITCH, M. P., 153, 240
National Cancer Study, 23
National Center for Health Statistics, 17, 22, 23–24, 27, 28, 29n, 30, 32, 34, 240–241
National Health Education Committee, 19–22, 32, 33, 34, 241
Neoplasms, malignant, data on, 22–23
Networks, social, 81, 164–165
NEUGARTEN, B., 85
NISBET, R., 88, 241
Nonidentity, and tension management, 108–109
Nonpatient, concept of, 40–41
Normality, concepts of, 49
Notifiable diseases, prevalence of, 26–27
NUCKOLLS, K. B., 166, 167, 241

O

OAKLEY, A., 149n, 241
OBEYESEKERE, G., 212, 241
OETTGEN, H. F., 104, 241
ORWELL, G., 73
OSTFELD, A. M., 166, 169, 237, 241–242
Overestimation, by vested interests, and morbidity data, 33–34
Overlap, of morbidity data, 32
Overload. See Load balance
OVESEY, L., 151, 238

P

Pain: as breakdown facet, 57–59; concept of, 58
PARKES, C. M., 166, 189, 202, 242
PARSONS, T., 50n, 203, 208, 211, 212, 242

Participation, sense of coherence related to, 155–156, 187, 189, 200, 205, 208, 212, 216

Pathogenesis: drawbacks of, 36–37; salutogenesis essential to, 45; ubiquity of, 12–14

Patient: concept of, 40–41; psychological needs of, 43–44; in relationship with health care system, 199–214

PATRICK, R., 171, 233

PAYKEL, E. S., 94–95, 245

PEARLIN, L. I., 172, 194, 242

PERLMUTER, L. C., 152–153, 242

Personality structure, basic, concept of, 149

PETRIE, A., 113, 242

Phase-specific crises, as psychosocial stressors, 84

PHILLIPS, D. P., 114, 242

Physical factors, as generalized resistance resources, 103–106

Plasticity, and tension management, 104

Potentiation, tension related to, 96

POWLES, J., 39n, 242

Predictability, sense of coherence related to, 126–127, 152, 187

Prognostic implication: as breakdown facet, 61–62; concept of, 62

Psychological variables: and health linked to sense of coherence, 171–175; impact of, 201; for sense of coherence, 137–142

R

RADLOFF, R., 95, 242

RAHE, R. H., 75, 81, 86, 110, 143, 176, 177, 178, 236, 237, 242–243

RAPOPORT, A., 122, 243

Rationality, as coping strategy, 112 113, 170

Religion, and tension management, 118

Respiratory conditions, chronic, data on, 24

Risk factor confusion, and morbidity data, 32

ROAZEN, P., 96, 243

ROESKE, N. A., 111, 243

Role-set complex, sense of coherence related to, 146, 147, 191

ROSE, R. M., 168, 233

ROSENBERG, B., 156, 231

ROSENMAN, R., 173–174

ROSENSTOCK, I. M., 100–101, 243

ROTTER, J. B., 152–153, 155, 158, 171, 243

ROUECHE, B., 26, 243

Routine encounters, impact of, on sense of coherence, 202–207

RUESCH, J., 171, 243

RUTSTEIN, D. D., 51, 243

S

Sacred modality, of doctor-patient relationship, 209, 212–213, 214, 215

SALBER, E. J., 42, 245

Salutogenesis: concept of, 12–13; as essential to pathogenesis, 45; evolution of perspective on, 1–11; implications of, for health care system, 198–219; model of, 182–197; significance of, 35–37, 226–227

SCHACHTEL, E. G., 108–109, 243

SCHEFF, T. J., 25, 243

Schizophrenia, social-structural sources of, 142, 161–162

SCHMALE, A. H., 137–138, 139, 162, 166, 235, 243, 244

SCHOOLER, C., 144, 194, 238, 242

SCHRÖDINGER, E., 78, 120, 243

SCHUR, M., 81, 132, 243

SCHWARTZ, H., 193n, 232

SCOTT, R. A., 59, 72, 112, 243–244

SEGALL, A., 3

Self-direction, sense of coherence related to, 144, 145, 146–147

SELIGMAN, M. E. P., 107, 137, 139–140, 141, 153, 154, 165–166, 172, 175, 179, 244

SELYE, H., 5, 74, 93, 94, 99, 105, 129, 180, 194, 196, 244

Sense of coherence. *See* Coherence,
   sense of
SHALIT, B., 110, 148, 244
SHAW, G. B., 157
SHEEHY, G., 88, 244
SHOHAM, I., 8, 162, 231
SHUVAL, J. T., 2, 43, 95, 244
SIMMEL, G., 88, 244
SIMON, W., 88–89, 244
Situational variables, and health
   linked to sense of coherence, 175–
   179
Social environment, and health
   linked to sense of coherence, 168
Social networks: experiences in, as
   psychosocial stressors, 81; and
   health linked to sense of coherence,
   164–165
Social relations, conflictual, as psy-
   chosocial stressor, 87–88
Social-role complexes, in salutogenic
   model, 191
Social-structural variables: and health
   linked to sense of coherence, 163–
   168; for sense of coherence, 142–
   148
Social supports: as generalized resistance resources, 114–117; and
   health linked to sense of coherence,
   166–168
Socialization, inadequate, as psychosocial stressor, 86,
SOLOMON, G. F., 181, 244
SOROCHAN, W. D., 68, 244
Specific resistance resources (SRRs),
   in salutogenic model, 193, 194
SPITZ, R., 140, 179
SROLE, L., 25, 244
STARR, P., 218, 244
Status integration, and health linked
   to sense of coherence, 166
STERLING, P., 39n, 235
STERNBACH, R. A., 57
Stress: defined, 93; in salutogenic
   model, 195–196; tension distinct
   from, 3, 10, 96, 180
Stressors: as absence of generalized
   resistance resources, 119–120;

avoidance of, 100–102; characteristics of, 71–73; defined, 72; on
   group level, 91–92; as objective or
   subjective, 73–76; perception of,
   72–73; psychosocial, 79–91; in
   salutogenic model, 192–193; tension and stress related to, 70–97;
   ubiquity of, 70, 76–91
Structural variables, and sense of
   coherence, 142–148, 163–168
Substitutability, and tension management, 119
SUSSER, M., 25–26, 47, 48–50, 59,
   244
Sweden, job complexity and control
   in, 148
SWEENEY, D. R., 137–138, 244
SYME, S. L., 66, 163–164, 167, 245
SZASZ, T., 25, 205, 245

                           T

TAEUBER, C., 68, 245
Tanala culture, and sense of co-
   herence, 150–151
Tension: character of, 92–97; de-
   fined, 94; stress distinct from, 3,
   10, 96, 180
Tension management: and avoidance
   of stressors, 100–102; concept of,
   3, 96; and generalized resistance
   resources, 98–122; in salutogenic
   model, 193–195
THACKER, S. B., 42, 245
THOMAS, L., 11, 121, 221–222, 223,
   224, 225, 226, 245
THOMAS, W. I., 113
TIGER, L., 82
TINLING, D. C., 137–138, 244
TOFFLER, A., 83, 245
TORFS, C. P., 66, 245
Traumatic situations, impact of, on
   sense of coherence, 200–202
TRILLING, L., 132–134
Type A behavior pattern, as psycho-
   logical variable, 174–175
TYROLER, H. A., 83, 171, 233, 245

U

Underestimation, and morbidity data, 33
Underload. *See* Load balance
Urban environment, and health linked to sense of coherence, 169
U.S. Department of Health, Education and Welfare, 34

V

Valuative-attitudinal factors, as generalized resistance resources, 110–114
VICKERS, G., 97, 245
Visual impairment, data on, 20–21
Voodoo death, and sense of coherence, 165–166

W

WEISENBERG, M., 57, 245
WEISSMAN, M. M., 94–95, 245
Well-being, health related to, 67–69
WERTHEIM, E. S., 107, 137, 140–141, 157, 245–246

WHITE, K. L., 16–17, 246
WILLIAMS, T. F., 16–17, 246
WINKELSTEIN, W., 15–16, 34, 246
Withdrawal, sense of coherence related to, 138–139, 166
WITHEY, S. B., 68, 229
WOHLWILL, J. F., 87, 246
WOLF, S., 75–76, 105, 169, 170, 246
WOLFF, H., 75, 79, 105, 169, 170, 237
Work, substantive complexity of, and sense of coherence, 144–145, 147, 148
World Health Organization (WHO), deficiencies of health definition by, 52–55

Y

YOUNG, A., 212, 213, 246
YOUNG, J. L., 23, 234

Z

ZETZEL, E. R., 96
ZOLA, I. K., 3, 17, 77, 238–239, 246